Getting the Mercury Out

Áine Ní Cheallaigh

Published by
Capsule Press
Beacon, NY

Published by Capsule Press, Beacon, NY
www.capsulepress.com

ISBN-13: 978-1461131779

ISBN-10: 1461131774

I

Silver or White?

This book is about getting the mercury out, so the best moment to start this story is when my exposure to mercury began. It was a Wednesday afternoon. If it had been any other day of the week, things might have turned out differently, but it happened to be a Wednesday, so this is how it went.

On this particular day, one of our teachers happened to be sick, so we had a free class. This was an Irish secondary school run by the Sisters of Mercy. For the nuns, 'free class' meant quiet supervised study time. We were in one of the science rooms, so my friends and I crowded our stools up to a bench near the back so we could have a whispered conversation. The topic at hand was my tooth. It had been aching on and off for a couple of weeks. Today was one of the worse days.

"You should go to the dentist," my friend Mairead said. "I went all last month. It was brilliant."

Dentistry didn't sound brilliant to me. I hadn't been for an appointment since I was little, but a few years back, I'd tagged along while an older sister had a tooth extracted. The word 'dentist' conjured up visions of soaking red handkerchiefs, and my mother scolding my sister, saying she brought it on herself by sticking her finger in the hole to see if the tooth was really gone.

"I don't want to get a tooth pulled. All that blood," I shivered.

"I got mine pulled and I didn't bleed at all," Mairead said. "But pulling one tooth is not enough. What you need is lots of brown in your teeth to get fillings."

She opened up her mouth and showed us the shiny silver surfaces on her molars.

"Fourteen fillings!" she said. "It took every Monday morning for a month. Do you know how much Maths I missed? Brilliant."

"Do you think I need fillings too?" I asked and opened my mouth wide.

"Oh definitely," she said. "Loads of brown."

"Mairead Considine and Áine Ní Cheallaigh! What on Earth are you doing?" the teacher demanded.

"Nothing, miss," we said, and took up our textbooks in a pretense of studying.

"Make sure you go to Dr. Whelan," Mairead whispered out of the side of her mouth. "He gives lots of fillings."

She wrote his phone number in the margin of my physics book. This was good. Dr. Whelan was our family dentist, the one who'd pulled my sister's tooth.

"Go during your worst class," Mairead said. "That's the time he'll take you every week."

My worst class was Irish with Miss Burke. She hated

me, I hated her. It was easier to take in the mornings, but on a Wednesday afternoon, right after lunch, it was torture to hear her droning on about ancient Irish literature. What made it worse this Wednesday was that my tooth really really hurt.

I raised my hand, excused myself and went down to the office, where the secretary made my appointment. I walked out of school, over to Dr. Whelan's office, climbed into his chair, got the aching tooth pulled, and then blithely made one of the worst decisions of my life.

"You're going to need eleven fillings," he said. "We can start right away. Do you want the silver ones or the white ones?"

"How many times will I have to come back?" I asked.

"Three," he said. "It's best to anaesthetize only one quadrant of the mouth at a time, it keeps you from drooling like an idiot."

"Great," I said. This was turning out exactly as planned.

"So silver or white?"

"What's the difference?" I asked.

"The white ones are more expensive."

I thought about my parents who were going to foot the bill for this whole escapade.

"Definitely silver," I said.

❧❦

It would have been very revealing if my health had spiraled down the drain right away. But that's not how mercury poisoning works. If I sit back now and scratch my head, it's not easy to come up with a definitive First Mercury Symptom. I loved secondary school for the first three years, but the tide turned and I hated it for years four and five. Did the fact that I had my amalgams placed at the beginning of my fourth year have anything to do with this?

It could have just been a big case of adolescent angst, compounded by difficult home circumstances. I was the seventh of eight children, not unusual for a Catholic family in rural Ireland in the 1980s. By the time I was finishing secondary school, it was just me and my younger sister living at home with my parents. My parents were tired out, uncommunicative, with nothing to give after decades of hard parenting. My younger sister was developmentally delayed because of a brain injury she had suffered during an epileptic seizure. It's easy to pin it on circumstances, but looking back, my joy and emotional resilience began to slowly drain away during those years.

At the age of 18, I left my rural home to go to college in Dublin. I chose Dublin because it was Ireland's largest city, and I wanted a fresh start in a place that was as different from the insular rural community I grew up in as possible.

City life suited me. I enjoyed the independence, being exposed to new ideas and getting free of the conservative

Catholic ideals I was brought up with. And yet, I was far from happy.

In my second year of college, I began to have stress-related breakdowns. Exam times often triggered huge anxiety and uncontrollable distress. I was a good student, far more knowledgeable than most of my classmates about many of the subjects we were being examined on, but I just couldn't handle my emotions and perform under stress.

In later years, when I learned about mercury toxicity, I read about how the first symptoms manifest as subtle emotional changes. Depression creeps in. There is an unwarranted sensitivity and irritability. Emotional reactions become less reasonable, even as the mercury toxic person insists that their reaction is a totally logical response to their circumstances.

That sums up my college days, and beyond, into my twenties. I sought out psychotherapy at the age of 19 and believed without question that the reason I was feeling awful so much of the time was because I had grown up in a dysfunctional family. There were plenty of reasons for me to feel like crap, top of the list being the fact that my parents had essentially left me to raise myself. They were busy struggling to care for my brain-injured younger sister whose case of epilepsy resisted all drug treatment, and whose behavior problems were off the charts. Why would there be any reason to look beyond that when searching for the cause of my emotional distress?

And yet, even now, I hear my therapist's voice in my head saying, Why does it have to be childhood trauma or mercury? Why so black and white? Can't it be a bit of both?

I have put a lot of thought into that question. If heavy metals weren't in the picture, would I have shaken off my childhood and lived a serene adult life, without the aid of therapy? The fact of the matter is, I don't know. I really don't. I know how emotionally stable I feel now that the mercury is gone. How can I tease out how much of that stability stems from a freedom from heavy metals, and how much is based on a hard-won foundation of emotional work I did during years of therapy? There is no way to ever know.

Mercury toxicity usually starts with emotional symptoms. Then a few years later, the physical symptoms arrive. When I left Ireland after college and moved to New York City, every week I put aside a good chunk of the money I earned as a nanny to pay for the best therapist I could find. I knew that I was emotionally delicate and this was the best way to spend my money. I didn't even consider spending a penny on health insurance. Why should I? I was as strong as an ox. All through my twenties, I didn't exercise, I ate a diet that was mostly made up of two main food groups, sugar and potatoes.

And yet I rarely fell ill. The only mild ailment I suffered from was chronic constipation. But I'd been like that since childhood, it was just the way I was. I basically saw myself as having an iron constitution.

But at the age of 27, I had an episode that made me change the way I viewed my health.

It started with a case of shin splints. I'd had these before, when I was very young. They are pains felt in the lower leg bones, often dismissed as 'growing pains.' When I was a little girl, I would cry myself to sleep at night from the pain. And now, mysteriously, they were back. I looked them up online, and found that there was no known cause or cure, I should just take painkillers and wait for them to pass.

A few days later, I experienced an episode of rectal discomfort, and searching the internet again, I learned that this was what a hemorrhoid was. Yuck. WebMD told me everything I needed to know to make it all right again—more fiber in my diet and Preparation H. Was I in my late twenties or my late sixties? I went to Duane Reade and bought a bunch of old-lady supplies.

The next morning, I got a nasty surprise when I looked at my face in the mirror. The area around my jaw was all swollen. It wasn't red, it didn't hurt, and it just looked like I was wearing a fat suit on the lower half of my face. What the hell? I went back to WebMD and learned that I had parotiditis, an infection of the salivary glands more commonly known as the mumps.

I had no energy that week. WebMD told me that there wasn't a lot I could do to treat parotiditis, except make sure my saliva kept flowing by sucking on lemon drops. I got dressed and walked slowly, very slowly back to the same Duane Reade and got my lemon drops. When I got back in bed, I lay there wondering what I'd done to make my health collapse. What would happen next? Was there anything I could do to prevent it?

৵৶৽

Over the next year, I worked, I hung out with my girl-friend, I spent a lot of my spare time writing, and I also kept one eye on my health. It seemed like there was always some weird niggling health mystery I had to solve. During this time, my girlfriend and I found an apartment together in Brooklyn, and something in the air of that apartment seemed to bother me. I developed cracked sores in the corners of my mouth. WebMD said they were caused by a fungus, and I cleared them up using an over-the-counter antifungal that had the attractive label 'jock itch cream.' I bought a humidifier, and that seemed to help too. I also made sure that my fiber intake was high so that my hemorrhoid wouldn't recur.

I had a good friend called Margaret who was in my writing group. She, too, had emigrated from the other side of the pond, so we had a lot in common. She was an English professor, Fulbright scholar, and dove deep into researching whatever her current area of interest was.

Her health had been the target of her laser-like focus recently. She had gone to the doctor with stomach complaints, and learned that she had ulcerative colitis. The doctor's proposed treatment plan was to cut out the ulcerated part of her intestine.

"Isn't that insane?" she asked us at our writing group meeting. "Who in their right mind would go straight to surgery as a first step? Do you know how many alternative treatments there are for colitis?"

I didn't, but with my little forays into WebMD and googling my symptoms, I could guess that there were a lot.

Margaret, of course, rejected the doctor's offer to cut the colitis out, and chose an alternative route. She saw a nutritionist who put her on a diet that seemed to consist of nothing more than rice, steamed chicken and kale. She also went for regular colonic irrigation sessions.

"The supplements are important too," she explained.

"What," I asked, "Like a multivitamin?"

"No," she said. "That whole 'Recommended Daily Amount' thing is a fraud. Do you know how much magnesium your body actually needs? You need far more than they can fit in one pill. You have to take them separately to get enough. And my nutritionist says they have to be the high quality ones or you won't absorb them. He won't let me buy the cheap ones."

"He sounds really strict," I said.

"Yeah, he's a bit of a Nazi alright," she shrugged. "But the fact that he's kinda crazy doesn't mean it won't work."

Margaret threw herself into her cure. It spilled over into her creative work, and at the writing group we read a humorous and thoughtful essay about the experience of going for a first colonic session. I figured the alternative healing world was full of crazies, selling potions and powders that didn't really work. But watching Margaret's story evolve, my position began to shift. Yes, the alternative healing world was full of crazies. That was absolutely true. They didn't seem to care that the things they said often contradicted basic laws of physics and chemistry. (People could be healed at a distance, thoughts could turn into molecules.) But there was something in there. After a few months on her chicken and kale diet Margaret was cured. It really didn't matter if her nutritionist guy was crackers, what he told her had saved her from surgery. It had really worked.

At this point, at the age of 30, I was by no means sick, but I wasn't exactly well either. I was intrigued by the possibilities presented by alternative healing.

"Given the trash that's in the standard American diet," Margaret said, "Is it any surprise that everyone's health crashes by the age of 30? We weren't designed to be eating like this!"

14

Hearing that I suffered from constipation, she tried to sell me on the idea of colonics.

"It's not gross at all," she said. "My guy is really respectful, he has excellent boundaries. He's pretty exclusive, but I can get you an appointment."

I could get behind a lot of what she was saying, but didn't want to go down that extreme road. And I definitely didn't want to have to carry a thermos of chicken and kale with me everywhere I went. My younger sister had been on a special diet. After years of every doctor in Ireland filling her up with doses of drugs that would have stopped a horse from having a seizure, she still had hundreds of petit mals by day, and frequent grand mals while she slept. The only thing that had worked was a treatment called the Ketogenic Diet, an extremely low carb, high fat diet that had cured her epilepsy for good.

Living on a hideously restricted diet like lettuce, tomatoes and coconut oil was worth it for extreme cases. But I was not an extreme case of anything, I was just curious. I wasn't going to go to those lengths, but I began to wonder if a small dietary change might reverse the downward trend in my health. The latest new symptom I'd noticed was moments of woozy lightheadedness and dark patches in my vision if I stood up too suddenly after I ate. WebMD told me that this kind of low blood pressure was a common sign of aging, and I should take care when I stood up after a meal, or I might fall and break a hip.

Were the alternative people right? Had I brought on premature aging through a diet of trash and sugar? I was ready to find out.

I researched online and found a book called *The Diet Cure*. The author seemed pretty grounded in reality and science, and the diet plan wasn't too extreme. No sugar in any form, lots of fresh vegetables, and protein with each meal to keep blood sugar steady. There were healthy snacks like nuts and fruit smoothies. It sounded like an ideal way to increase my overall health.

The author recommended going on the diet all at once, and using amino acids and other supplements to curb sugar cravings and ameliorate any detox symptoms that might arise in the few days of transition. I was intrigued by the amino acids. Tyrosine was supposedly going to give me more energy. Glutamine was going to help my blood sugar, and also heal my colon. I went to the vitamin store and got my supplements and some whey protein powder for my smoothies. Then I went to the health food store and filled my basket with organic vegetables. And the experiment began.

Even today, after all I've learned, I'm not sure why it went so terribly wrong. Back then, I didn't understand that I have the kind of metabolism that responds strongly to supplements even in tiny doses. On the first day of my new regimen, I went to the Y to work out—part of my new healthy lifestyle. I took some tyrosine for energy and I was off. The stationary bicycle had a feature that showed my heart rate as I exercised, and I saw that I was supposed to get it up to about 150 beats per minute to be in the target zone. I pedaled fast to get it up there, and it responded, climbing quickly up to 120, then 135, then 160. I slowed down, but the numbers kept climbing, 172 then 185.

I looked at the chart. This was way too high. My maximum heart rate was supposed to be 190. I stopped pedaling altogether, and sat there listening to the staccato hammering of my heart in my ears, my eyes glued to the heart rate display: 201, 202. I started to panic and let go of the bar that was sensing my heart rate. I tried to calm down by focusing on just breathing and staying upright on the bike. What had I done to myself? After a few minutes, I touched the bar again, 185 and falling.

When I got home I googled 'tyrosine side effects' and learned that heart palpitations and rapid heartbeat could occur in sensitive individuals. It was easy enough to stop taking the tyrosine, but that was just the start of my troubles.

The next day, I was out shopping, browsing in the health food store, when I suddenly began to feel flushed and sweaty. My throat became dry and I felt dizzy, like I might pass out. I abandoned my basket and got out into the fresh air. After resting a while, I was able to make it home, but I was badly shaken by the incident. Was the detox phase really supposed to be this bad? I read up more about blood sugar and how it was important not to let it dip too low. I made sure I ate at least every two hours, but things kept getting worse.

The flushing-sweating-dizzy moment was not an isolated incident. Over the next few days, they increased in frequency until I was having them every couple of hours. I also began to notice a burning feeling in my colon, especially when I lay down at night to go to sleep. Worried, I abandoned the whole Diet Cure regimen, except for one exception. I didn't go back to eating sugar. It had been such a big deal to give it up, I had read so much about how bad it was for my health. Now that I apparently had some kind of blood sugar problem, the last thing I wanted was to go back to eating something that would make it worse.

Stopping the Diet Cure improved things considerably, but overall, I was now in worse condition than when I'd begun it. The facial flushing didn't entirely go away. It happened like clockwork every day at about 7pm, no matter what I ate.

Even now, I'm not sure what that was, or why the Diet Cure screwed me up so badly. I think a part of it was the sudden nature of the changes I made. My sensitive metal toxic system was balanced on a knife-edge of functionality. A number of changes thrown at it all at once toppled it. I also know now that mercury was impairing the function of my adrenals—low blood sugar and low blood pressure are big indicators of adrenal fatigue, and are common symptom of mercury toxicity. And I also think that taking in more protein than I was used to shifted my pH in the acidic direction, something that was exacerbated by my generally acidic state caused by my lead toxicity. Not to mention the strain heavy metals were putting on my liver.

But of course, at the time, I had no idea that I had to take into account an underlying case of heavy metal poisoning. I thought that my bad diet had brought about my ill health, so of course I threw myself into the search for the perfect diet. If food had gotten me into this mess, it was going to get me out of it.

Increasing my protein had gotten me in trouble with the Diet Cure, so I tried eating very little protein for a while. That didn't go well. I tried the food combining diet, where meats and grains were eaten at separate meals, but this didn't seem to work for me either. All through that whole winter, my face flushed every day, and I suffered terribly from the cold. If I didn't eat right away when I woke up in the morning, I would fall apart and start to cry. I read more about hypoglycemia online, and got a book about diabetes from the library.

The conventional wisdom seemed to be that a case of hypoglycemia could easily develop into full-blown diabetes. I worried about this. My mother had had gestational diabetes when she was pregnant with me and my sister, and had developed type 2 diabetes when I was a teenager.

Was there any way that I could stop this slide? Did I have some kind of genetic defect in my pancreas?

By springtime, I had started taking chromium to keep my blood sugar steady, a multivitamin and calcium for general health, and had settled on my version of the hypoglycemic diet. I didn't eat sugar, but I still ate fresh fruit. I ate six times a day to keep my blood sugar even, a chore I despised. Why did I have to be the freak who had to carry snacks everywhere they went, and ate by the clock? It seemed that every new food I tried caused problems. When I thought I'd found a good diabetic energy bar that would keep my blood sugar up, I'd find that it worsened my constipation and caused my hemorrhoid to rip open and bleed. I was eating an extremely healthy diet by normal standards, and yet my health wasn't getting any better. My face wouldn't stop flushing at 7pm despite all my work. My girlfriend didn't like it.

"I think it's time you went to the doctor," she said.

I really was not excited by the whole idea of doctors. I'd spent my childhood watching them trying to cure my sister's epilepsy and failing miserably.

"I don't have insurance," I said.

"You can go the gay and lesbian clinic," she countered. "They have a sliding scale."

"What good will it do me?" I asked. "Did doctors help Margaret?"

"They diagnosed her," she said. "They can run tests and diagnose you if there's something really wrong."

She had hit a nerve. I was doing everything I could to feel better, but I clearly wasn't well. When I spoke to Margaret about it, she said, *You're still detoxing.* But I didn't believe her. This wasn't normal. There had to be something causing this.

"Okay," I said. "But just to find out what's behind all this. I'm not taking any drugs."

I made sure I ate before I went in for my 7pm appointment. Even so, I could still feel my face flushing a little as I explained my symptoms to the doctor.

"Do you know what could cause all these symptoms?" I asked her.

"You're on the hypoglycemic diet now?" she asked.

"Yes."

"And you feel better on it?"

"Yes," I said.

"Well then, let's give you a tentative diagnosis of hypoglycemia." She turned and typed it into my file on the computer. "We'll take some blood, and if anything unusual comes up, we'll take it from there."

I got a jolly message from her on my answering machine a few days later.

"We got your blood work back, your liver enzymes are a little elevated, but that doesn't mean anything. Everything else is totally normal, nothing to worry about. Just continue with the hypoglycemic diet if it makes you feel better."

That was it? I'd paid hundreds of dollars for her to

parrot back to me that I thought I had hypoglycemia? What a waste of time and money.

Over the next year or so I kept scrambling around, trying different supplements, and reading reading reading. I tried different fiber supplements that people online swore by for constipation, but gave up on them when I developed an allergy to one called psyllium. Besides my customary two days of PMS where my brain went missing, and the hefty menstrual cramps I usually had, I now was starting to get symptoms in the middle of my cycle. I would get cranky and emotional for no reason.

Two years after my first health crisis with the mumps and the first appearance of my hemorrhoid, I was still struggling. Despite everything, I was still constipated, my hemorrhoid bled regularly. The burning feeling in my colon came and went. And my face still sometimes flushed even though I was on the healthiest diet I could possibly come up with. What was the point of working so hard on this if it didn't make me feel better? Was my case so hard to crack?

I took my troubles to Dr. Margaret. I had tried everything else. I was ready to hear what she had to say.

First I described my symptoms, then I described my diet. Then she asked about my supplements.

"Calcium you say?" she asked. "And how much

magnesium?"

"None," I said. "Unless it's in my multivitamin."

"Oh dear," she said. "No wonder you're constipated. Oh you poor thing. Calcium will stop you right up. You need lots of magnesium to make you go."

"Oh, okay." This sounded good.

"It will help with an acidic colon too," she added. "That's the burning feeling. Have you tested your pH?"

"Nope."

"Okay, order the test strips online, and read up about the acid/alkaline diet. All meat and most grains are acidic, but millet is really good. I'd give that a shot."

"I will," I said. "Thanks."

"And one more thing. Learn about your adrenals. Low blood sugar isn't about your pancreas. It's your adrenals."

I ordered a book called *Adrenal Fatigue: The 21st Century Stress Syndrome* by James Wilson. And there it was. The answer to the question my doctor was stumped by. What caused hypoglycemia? The answer was adrenal fatigue. And this was caused by stress, allergies, our toxic modern environment and bad diet. One of the supplements Wilson recommended was magnesium, and suddenly there were references to it everywhere I went. I even found a whole book about it on the shelf at my local Barnes and Noble called *The Magnesium Miracle*.

And indeed it was a miracle. As soon as I added magnesium to my supplement regimen, the tide began to turn. Instead of trying desperately to keep my head above water, I was slowly and surely making progress. Everything I tried now seemed to really work. The acid/alkaline diet cleared up my burning colon. Baking soda enemas cleared up my hemorrhoid problems. Thanks to magnesium, I was no longer constipated, and best of all, it lifted my mood, and I began to feel hope for my future. Instead of feeling like I was on the fast track to old age, I felt in control of my destiny. By cleaning up my diet and taking the right supplements, I had fixed all my problems. And if any new ones cropped up, I could always call Dr. Margaret.

"I have a spot on my breast," I told her one day. "It's like a freckle, but paler, and—"

"Don't worry," she said. "It's not skin cancer. I get it too. It's a fungus called tinea versicolor. A couple of days of antifungal cream from the drugstore will fix it up."

"Jock itch cream?" I asked, remembering the fungus in the corners of my mouth.

"That's the one. You might feel a bit cruddy the day after you first use it as the fungus dies off."

A few weeks later, she recommended the supplement Ginkgo Biloba for a painful varicose vein that had suddenly appeared running down the inside of my left leg. I was grateful that Margaret was seven or eight years older than I was. By the time anything came up for me, Margaret had encountered it already. I felt like she was an alternate version of me in the future, encountering the problems I would face, and lighting my path by doing all the research.

The Ginkgo made the varicose vein go away, and also had the wonderful side effect of sharpening my brain function. Two weeks into taking it, I was sitting around at work, waiting for the kids I babysat to finish their snack so I could take them to the playground. Their father was drinking coffee nearby, doing the New York Times crossword.

"Is it hard?" I asked. "I've never done it."

"Want to give it a shot?"

I nodded.

"Empty," he read. "Beginning with a 'v'."

"Void," I said.

"No, seven letters."

"Oh 'vacuous' then," I said.

"Right," he said, penciling it in. "Now how about 'coral producers'—"

"Polyps," I said.

"—with a y in the middle. Yeah, that looks good."

On we went, my Ginkgo enhanced brain crackling with all the right answers. By the time I had finished it, I could see a bemused look on his face, like, Who knew the babysitter was so smart?

It was wonderful to feel so good. I was getting compliments on my looks too. In the year since I'd done the Diet

Cure, I hadn't gone back to eating sugar, and I had slowly and steadily dropped 20lbs. I was now below 150lbs for the first time since I was a teenager, and was bang in the middle of the ideal Body Mass Index chart for a person my height. It felt great.

Things weren't perfect. I often paid a hefty price if I strayed from the eating schedule or set of foods I knew went down well. And I still had weird things crop up. One day I had a bit of a sore throat, and looked in the mirror to see a little white stone emerging from my left tonsil. And so I went online and learned all about Tonsil Stones, little white masses that popped out of some people's tonsils for no apparent reason. After some nasty headaches, I learned that I was reacting badly to MSG. And finding the right foods when I was traveling or eating out was always a bit dicey. But on the whole, life was quite pleasant and manageable.

And then Margaret found a lump in her breast. The official diagnosis was DCIS, at the earliest stage a breast cancer could be at. But the doctor wanted to schedule her for surgery later that week. She explained the whole thing when we met for lunch at our favorite health food restaurant.

"After the surgery, your nipple is completely gone," she said. "So they tattoo on a fake one. Barbaric. And this man has the gall to tell me that if I have a kid, I'll be able to breastfeed fine with one breast. What does he know about breastfeeding?"

"So you're not going to go for surgery?" I asked.

"No!" she said. "Do you know how many alternative treatments for cancer there are out there?"

I smiled.

"Lots?"

She took a book out of her bag and handed it to me. It was called *The Cure for All Cancers* by Hulda Clark.

"Doctors say that cancer has no known cause," she said. "It's just something that happens. Well it's just not true."

"What causes it?" I asked.

"Toxins," she said. "They're everywhere. Sodium laurel sulfate in your shampoo. Mercury in your teeth. Formaldehyde in your carpets. And plastic plastic everywhere."

"Plastic causes cancer?" I said.

"I'm removing every single toxic substance from my apartment," she said. "My mattress, my pillows, shampoos, cleaners, makeup, aluminium pans. I've filled ten garbage bags already and I'm not done yet. The place is almost empty."

"Holy shit."

"And that's just phase one. Next comes the cleansing."

She described the liver flushes and juice fasts and parasite cleanses that would free her body of its toxic burden, and allow it to kill the cancer on its own.

"It should take about six months," she said.

"And if it doesn't work, are you going to go back to the doctor for surgery?" I asked.

"It's going to work," she said. "None of my friends want to hear this. Everyone's trying to convince me to go back to the doctor. They hear the 'c' word and it scares the shit out of them. I need people who can support me through this."

"I will," I said.

But I was scared too. Scared for Margaret and scared for myself. On my way home, I stopped at Barnes and Noble and found *The Cure for All Cancers* on the shelf. Beside it was Hulda Clark's even more extravagantly titled *The Cure for All Diseases*. That was the one I picked up and brought home. I wasn't reading this just to be supportive of Margaret. I was reading this for me.

I felt that I was following in Margaret's health footsteps. She had colitis, I had a burning colon. She had tinea versicolor, I had tinea versicolor. She was constipated, I was constipated. She had varicose veins, I had varicose veins. Everything I had, she'd had already. And now she had cancer. At the age of 38. Just seven more years until I'd get it too. Unless I did something right now to prevent it.

I went straight home and dove into *The Cure for All Diseases*. There were lists of conditions, but I couldn't figure out which one I had. What exactly was I trying to cure? It didn't matter. The cure for all of them was the same. Removing the toxins from your life, killing parasites, flushing your liver. I was disappointed to read that liver flushes weren't recommended if you had any silver fillings in your mouth. These fillings contained mercury, and it was better to get the mercury out before attempting a liver flush. But even with mercury in your mouth, it was still fine to kill parasites. I was in the middle of writing down a shopping list for Radio Shack when my girlfriend came home.

"What are you doing?" she asked.

I explained that I was preparing to assemble a simple electric device called a zapper which, if tuned to the correct frequency, could kill the hidden parasites in my body and prevent cancer.

"Ooookaay," she said. "Where did you get this idea?"

I told her about my lunch with Margaret, explained about the toxins and the plastics and the liver flushes, and showed her *The Cure for All Diseases.*

"Oh sweetheart," she said. "There is no cure for all diseases. If there was, we would have heard about it on the news. This person is a quack. There are no parasites hidden inside people. It's all just crazy talk."

"It is?" I asked.

"It's time to step away from the book," she said. "And join the rest of us back in the real world."

"Okay," I said, beginning to cry. "But is Margaret going to be all right?"

"She has stage zero cancer," my girlfriend said, "Even if it grows a little while she's trying an alternative cure, it's still okay. She can go for surgery later, she has plenty of time. There's no way this cancer will kill her. She'll really be okay."

৶৯৶

Over the next couple of months, we watched the already-slim Margaret turn a bit skeletal. She wasn't really eating much food. She had her own juicer, and was living mostly on vegetable juice. She showed me how it worked. Carrots and celery went in the top, got mashed against some spinning blades. Juice came out one end, and pulp came out the back. I took a sip and it tasted pretty good.

"Sometimes I get so hungry," she said. "I eat the pulp too."

Every now and then, especially after an intense bout of cleansing with bentonite clay, she would report, "I think the lump is shrinking."

We cheered her on, encouraged her and brought her bags of organic vegetables, but wondered if the lump was shrinking just because the rest of her was shrinking too.

But at the end of three months, she announced that the cleanse had been a success. The lump was gone. She began to eat regular food, filled out again to her normal size, and to this day, five years later, remains cancer free.

Watching this not only made me a believer, but convinced my girlfriend too. We bought a juicer and occasionally had mini-fasts where we juiced and ate raw food for a few days. My girlfriend didn't really want to take it further than that, her health wasn't delicate like mine. But I was intrigued by the cleanses Margaret had done.

When Margaret had done the parasite cleanse, it had yielded a number of foot-long tapeworms. I tried the parasite cleanse too, but with less dramatic results. I just got tired and constipated and sometimes passed weird pink rubbery-looking lumps in my poop.

"Um, how do you know your parasite cleanse is, uh, successful?" I asked Margaret one day. "Do the tapeworms sometimes come out in little pieces?"

"Nope," Margaret said. "Believe me, you'll know when it happens. You'll look in the toilet bowl and say, "What the hell is that?'"

I kept up with the parasite cleanse, a tincture of black walnut, wormwood, and cloves that I had to take three times a day for three weeks, and still nothing happened. It just wore out my liver. And the more I learned about my liver, the more I was convinced I'd benefit from a liver flush. Chronic constipation and bad digestion were linked with low bile flow, and I wanted to clear the blockages out of my liver and get the bile moving freely.

The only thing standing between me and some serious liver flushing was the fact that I had amalgam fillings. Hulda Clark said that liver flushes shouldn't be attempted until the mercury was all gone. I ran this past Margaret.

"Yeah, the fillings have to go," Margaret said. "It's not smart to get them done while you're shrinking a lump, because it stirs up mercury. But they're next on the list for me."

She gave me the number of the dentist she planned to use, a holistic dentist that her colonic guy recommended.

"She uses all the precautions," Margaret said. "And guides you through the detox with all the right supplements. It's quite dangerous to go to a regular dentist and start drilling them out."

I took the number and tucked it away in a safe place. Getting my fillings done wasn't a trivial matter. I was going to do my homework before I took the plunge.

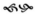

There were a lot of different herbs and supplements recommended online for mercury detox. As I scanned all the different regimens, I made a list of the supplements that were recommended most often: Vitamin C, MSM, NAC, garlic, chlorella, and zinc.

There was a lot of talk online about the dangers of mercury, but the people who seemed to get sick during amalgam removal were people whose health was in pretty poor shape to start with. I was glad I was doing this while I was still young, before mercury'd had a chance to mess with my health. As usual, the science behind the alternative health advice sounded a bit made up, so I was glad to stumble across a scientific paper investigating the effects of amalgam removal on blood mercury levels.

The paper described how a number of people had their blood mercury levels tested before amalgam removal, and then at regular intervals in the year that followed. The study showed that amalgam removal raised blood levels of mercury directly after amalgam removal, but that by the time a year had passed, it had fallen down to the level of an average person. This paper reassured me. Even if getting my fillings out made me a little bit sick, it would all have died away by the time a year had passed.

I called Margaret's dentist and made an appointment.

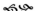

Her office was on the Upper West Side, your basic ground-floor practice with its own entrance. Receptionist, waiting room, bathroom, and then the hallway leading down to the rooms where the action happened. My first appointment was intake and x-rays, and a blood test to make sure that I wasn't allergic to the material my new white fillings were going to be made of. This stuff was called 'composite' and was a lot cheaper than gold or any of the other non-toxic filling materials.

Since she was a holistic dentist, she of course had an intake form that was pages long, asking me to describe my health in detail. I felt pretty smug saying that my only problem was hypoglycemia, but my diet had it under control. Then after thinking about it for a bit, I ticked another box called 'Food Allergies.' That about summed up the fact that a lot of the new foods I tried didn't go down well, even though I wasn't sure exactly what the problem ingredient was.

I handed my form over the receptionist.

"Áine Ní Cheallaigh," she read, pronouncing it perfectly: *Awn-ya Nee Kallig.* This was the first time since I'd arrived in New York that someone had pronounced my name correctly right off the bat.

"You're Irish," I said, and told her what county I was from. Apparently she had just arrived in New York, and wasn't very impressed with the New Yorkers who were her boss's clients.

"Sure aren't they're bonkers, every last one of them," she rolled her eyes. "They all have these delusions that their fillings are poisoning them. They call here and say, 'I need to get my fillings out because they're giving me headaches.' Headaches, I ask you! Sure couldn't anything give you a headache! Absolutely bonkers!"

I extracted myself quickly and went back to the waiting room, thinking, I'm one of those bonkers clients too. Don't assume I agree with you just because I'm Irish.

my health. I was feeling more tired than usual, but not tired enough to limit my usual activities. I went to work, and even took up the challenge of writing a whole novel in a month in my spare time. I won the challenge easily, but kept noticing a drain on my energy that had started with my first amalgam removal appointment.

Another mercury symptom reared its ugly head during this time. My hemorrhoid, which had been totally healed up ever since I'd started taking magnesium, opened up and started to bleed quite copiously. Any time it had bothered me before, it had only bled during bowel movements, but now a little bit of blood was always seeping out of my rectum. My period arrived, much heavier, and with worse PMS and cramps than usual. I began to wonder how much blood loss was too much.

Mercury seemed to be having a negative effect on my whole digestive system. I often felt mildly nauseated, and had odd aches and pains in my gut. I wondered if there was anything I could do about any of this. Were the detox supplements I was taking making things worse?

I was taking MSM, vitamin C, chlorella and zinc. This was besides my regular regimen of chromium, magnesium, glutamine and ginkgo biloba.

First I axed the vitamin C because I read online that large doses of vitamin C acted as a blood thinner. Stopping it made the bleeding much more manageable, I now only bled during bowel movements. Next, I cut out the chlorella, which seemed to help too. Zinc was next to go.

As soon as I stopped taking it, the nausea disappeared.

The following week, I had my fourth and final amalgam removal appointment. Each appointment had been easier than the one before. I wasn't dreading it at all. In fact, I was very much looking forward to all the fillings being gone. Finally, I would be able to chew, floss and drink hot liquids without thinking about how much mercury was being released into my system.

"I'm going to take one more look at your blood," the dentist said when the drilling and filling was over.

During the course of the appointments, she had talked a bit about the blood testing method she used. It wasn't a conventional blood test, but rather an energy test where she held the sample of my blood in one hand, and held the substance to be tested in the other. She said that it worked just as well as a conventional blood test, and though it sounded nutty, I believed her.

"Your blood has mercury in it, which is to be expected," she said, when she came back into the room. "But it also has a much higher level of lead."

"Really?" I said. "Where would lead come from?"

"I don't know," she said. "Lead is in a lot of different things. But I can get you EDTA suppositories that will remove the lead from your system. I can order them, I'll give you a call when they come in."

I went home and googled sources of lead. Apparently it often was in enamel bathtubs or cookware. Some pottery glazes contained lead. I spent the next few days going around the house with the little lead testing stick I got at the hardware store. I swabbed every surface I could think of that might contain lead, from the dishes to the countertops to the inside of the microwave. They all came up negative.

I fretted about it at first. But then as the last traces of mercury faded from my system, and my health returned to normal, I just let it go. I decided not to go back to the dentist to pick up the EDTA suppositories. Messing around with more detox supplements really wasn't appealing. I stopped taking MSM, the last of the detox supplements, and put the whole heavy metal episode behind me.

❧❧

Of course the whole mercury episode was not behind me. There were many chapters to go before I could close the book on heavy metals, but I wasn't aware of that yet. I may have been done with mercury, but mercury was not done with me.

I didn't know, and nobody told me, that my years of exposure to amalgam meant I had a storehouse of mercury secreted away in the cells and organs of my body. My breath was the conduit that had, day in, day out, brought mercury vapor from my mouth down into my lungs. My bloodstream, greedily drinking in oxygen, had also taken on a cargo of mercury, and carried it all

41

over my internal terrain. On its way through my liver, my thyroid, my brain, my very cells, it had dropped molecules of mercury. And because mercury also blocked up the hatches that allowed metals to move out of cells, any mercury that got dropped inside a cell had a hard time getting out again.

But amalgam removal changed everything. My breath no longer brought steady doses of mercury into my system when I inhaled. My liver and kidneys were able to catch up. Over the next three months, they were able to clear my bloodstream of this dreaded toxin.

But scrubbing my bloodstream so clean meant that my cell walls got a bit of a spring cleaning too. Mercury that had been blocking the passage of metals in and out of cells was now gone. Metals were free to move in ways that they hadn't been in years.

And one of those metals was mercury.

Not all at once, but slowly and steadily, all the sleeping atoms of mercury that had been sitting quietly in my cells got the call. In increasing numbers, they flooded out of my cells, into my bloodstream, and did what heavy metals do—they caused havoc. Overwhelmed, my liver and kidneys could only excrete a small portion of them every day. And every day, more and more poured out of my cells to replace their excreted brothers.

Nothing could stop this rising tide. My blood mercury rose far beyond anything I had seen in my sixteen years of amalgam exposure. The organs that mercury targets: my brain, my liver, my adrenals, my thyroid, were screwed. And it went on and on and on.

This phenomenon is referred to as the 'Detox Roller-coaster Ride' or more descriptively, the 'Dump Phase.' The first signs of mercury being dumped into the blood-stream appear three to six months after the last amalgam is removed.

But first, there is the calm before the storm. Before the mercury hits the fan, the patient experiences an incredible reprieve from all their mercury symptoms. It's a beautiful thing. And it's the last glimpse of good health that they're going to see for a very very long time.

II

⊰❧

The Dump Phase

The week after I had my last amalgam removed, I decided to stop eating gluten for a while. After what the dentist had said about food allergies, I wanted to check and see if I had celiac disease like her. I wasn't 100% sure which packaged foods had gluten in them. Most ingredient lists didn't specify. So I just steered my choices towards the foods I usually ate that were naturally gluten free: millet, potatoes, sprouted grains, fruits and vegetables, peas and beans.

I didn't notice anything dramatic for the first few days. I didn't really think much about it until the fourth day, when I woke up feeling poorly. I had a headache and was in a bad mood. This was a kind of headache I often got. I hated it. It wasn't very painful, but no matter what I did, it was always there in the background, going on and on for hours. I'd never thought very hard about the cause of it before. But today, I wondered, could it possibly be gluten? Had I eaten some accidentally?

I went out into the kitchen and mentally retraced my eating steps from the day before.

Breakfast: millet, plain yoghurt, raisins, cinnamon. I pulled out the packages and looked. All of them were single ingredient foods. All clean.

Lunch: an avocado on Ezekiel sprouted bread. The avocado was obviously fine, but what about the bread? I took the loaf out the freezer and examined the ingredients list. The first ingredient on the list was Organic Sprouted Wheat. I'd picked up the little tidbit of information somewhere that if a grain was sprouted, it became gluten free, but was that actually true? Was this bread really gluten free?

I went online and quickly found out that I had unwittingly ingested gluten by eating this bread. I also learned that even if the bread had been gluten free, there was a good chance it had picked up some lingering gluten crumbs while sitting in the toaster.

Eureka.

I got my gluten free diet back on track, and my head felt clear and my mood sunny in the days that followed. It was a revelation. I decided I wouldn't make any more mistakes, and started educating myself by reading lists of safe foods and following the discussion boards at celiac. com.

Before my girlfriend and I went to the health food supermarket for our next weekly shopping trip, I purged the kitchen of glutenous foods that I knew that neither of us would ever eat. The energy bars sweetened with barley malt, the breaded fish sticks and chicken nuggets that my vegetarian girlfriend wouldn't touch. They filled up the garbage can, and I looked at them sadly. There was no going back. Celiac disease was a lifetime condition that couldn't be reversed.

"Goodbye forever," I said and closed the garbage can.

My girlfriend put her arm around me as I started to cry.

"You're being very brave," she said. "You're a good girl."

Later, walking home from the store, I perked up considerably. I had given myself permission to buy six different kinds of gluten free cookies. My health mystery was solved. Gluten was the real culprit, not sugar. So I was reaching into my shopping bag and having a little sugar party to celebrate.

"These lemon wafers are pretty good," I said, offering a bite to my girlfriend.

"Definitely edible," she said.

"Uck, but these chocolate chip ones are terrible," I said. "Want to try?"

"When you put it like that," she said. "No thanks."

As the days and weeks passed, I felt better and better. My head was clear, my digestion was good, my mood was great, I had buckets of physical and emotional stamina. It was clear that gluten had somehow been at the root of all my health problems.

Researching more, I read that people on the gluten free diet often ended up low on B vitamins because gluten grains were the main source of them in the human diet. I supplemented with a B complex for a couple of weeks, but the supplement caused a terrible stiffness and pain to build up in the left side of my neck. I stopped taking it and it went away. I decided to stop taking all of my other supplements too. Why was I taking them? I was healthy now. All I needed was the gluten free diet, and I would be perfectly healthy forever.

Two months into the gluten free diet, I was healthier than I'd ever been. I was able to eat anything I wanted, as long as it was gluten free. I ate dessert daily, doing my best to make up for those two years I went without sugar. Hypoglycemia was a thing of the past. And best of all, my mood was calm and even. My girlfriend remarked on it to all our friends.

"How did you do it?" they asked.

"I went to the dentist to get my fillings out," I always began. I liked to fool around and imply that it was some kind of mercury filling removal miracle story. But I always explained what really happened.

"My dentist has celiac disease," I said. "And when I said I had food allergies, she told me to try the gluten free diet. And I did. And I found out I'm totally allergic!"

It didn't occur to me for one second that mercury had anything to do with it. It didn't even cross my mind that there was a connection between amalgam removal and my disappearing symptoms. When I ate gluten free, I felt great. If I ate some gluten accidentally, I felt terrible. Case closed.

∽§∾

I didn't feel that I really needed to, but since it had been the point of this whole exercise of getting my amalgams out, I went ahead and planned my first Hulda Clark liver flush. I took a booster dose of the parasite killer the night before I began. It had never done anything for me before except make me tired. But this dose was recommended in the liver flush instructions, so I dutifully took it. And right before my first liver flush began, I surprised myself greatly by pooping out an 8 inch long tapeworm. I knew that it was impossible to pass a live worm, but it was still an alarming sight.

Wow! I thought. *Wow! This thing was living inside me! Holy shit!*

I grabbed the cordless phone, brought it into the bathroom and called Margaret.

"It's not flat looking," I said, poking at it with a chopstick in the toilet bowl. "Are you sure it's a tapeworm?"

"Does it basically look like a very long earthworm?" she asked.

"Yup," I said.

"Well that's what certain kinds of tapeworms look like," she said. "Google 'images of fish tapeworms' and you'll see. Anyway, congratulations on your successful cleanse!"

The long-awaited liver flush happened the next day. The instructions on the Hulda Clark website said that I should expect to feel nauseous. This made me a little nervous. How bad was this going to be? At the same time, I was excited. This Hulda Clark stuff really worked. Even if the cleanse was a bit rough, the results would be worth it. All the gunk in my liver was going to get cleaned out.

I followed the instructions in Hulda Clark's book and fasted after lunch and then began to drink doses of Epsom salts dissolved in water. The Epsom salts solution tasted absolutely terrible, it was very hard to get it down. By the time I had to take my second dose, I was feeling quite queasy. Was this really worth it? Right before bed, I downed the drink that would make my liver expel stones: half a cup of olive oil mixed with half a cup of grapefruit juice. It didn't taste anywhere near as bad as the Epsom salts.

I fell asleep, woke up briefly during the night feeling nauseated, and the next morning, woke up and started pooping stones. Some were pink and rubbery, like the ones I'd seen during previous parasite cleanses. Some were pea green, but most of them were tan. I peered at them as they floated in the toilet bowl. Here they were, the famous liver stones that I'd read so much about. Left inside they body, they congested the liver and filled up the gall bladder. When they got infected, people needed gall bladder surgery. I was proud that I had gotten them out. It was just a few dozen stones, some of them just an eighth of an inch in diameter, others up to half an inch.

Hulda Clark said that one liver flush would improve health temporarily, but multiple flushes were necessary for permanent change. Passing a total of two thousand stones was apparently the benchmark. I wrote down 87 in my notebook, and wondered what kind of temporary improvements I'd notice.

◈

Eating at home on the gluten free diet was a breeze. It was only eating out that presented a challenge, but since we lived in New York City, it really wasn't that much of a big deal. It wasn't very difficult to go online and scope out safe places to eat in most neighborhoods. They didn't like to make a big deal about it—probably because 'gluten free' sounded too much like 'health food'— but lots of restaurants had separate gluten free menus if you asked. Their kitchen staff had been trained to avoid accidental contamination of food with gluten, and you could rest assured that they weren't cutting up your rice crust pizza on the same cutting board they used for the wheat ones.

But we weren't going to be in New York City for long. My girlfriend and I were finally taking the plunge and moving out of the city. We were going to be living in a very rural area near where my girlfriend's father lived. Its remoteness was offset somewhat by the fact that the train to New York City was a two-minute walk from our house. My girlfriend was going to keep her job and commute into the city, but I quit my job as a nanny and was looking for a new one upstate.

It was a big transition, so to help me out while I found my feet in my new community, I decided to go back to see my old therapist for a while. She had been very helpful when I'd first moved to New York City, helping me sort out my feelings about my dysfunctional family back in Ireland, and giving me permission to discover my true voice and creativity. I'd stopped seeing her for a couple of years because I felt that I got more out of working on my physical rather than my emotional health. But this was a good time to rekindle a connection with someone who knew me so thoroughly.

At our first session back, there was a lot of catch-up. We finally made it up to recent events: having a real house with a real garden where we could grow our own vegetables, how great getting on the gluten free diet had been, and the successful liver cleanse.

"I mean, it would have been better if I'd gotten out hundreds of stones," I said. "My ultimate goal is two thousand. But I was pretty happy."

Her brow creased.

"I don't understand," she said. "All of these stones. Don't they overflow the toilet bowl?"

I smiled and remembered who I was talking to. This was the woman I'd caught sneaking a cigarette out on the sidewalk before one of our sessions, someone who hadn't understood what I meant when I said I was trying a 'high fiber diet.'

I backed up and explained some more. For good

measure, I threw in a graphic description of my friend the tapeworm.

"Oy vey is mir," she said. "It must make such a difference not to have a worm inside you anymore."

I smiled and nodded, but the reality was that I wasn't really feeling much better. The truth was that I'd begun to feel a little bit worse.

I had been to a Passover Seder the week before and had been delighted to see that our host had baked a flourless chocolate cake. This was an intensely rich and yummy gluten free treat, and I had eaten practically half of it all by myself.

The next day, I was very disappointed to find that my digestive system could not handle that much chocolate. My hemorrhoid, which had been dormant since amalgam removal, began to bleed again. I had thought that being on the gluten free diet meant that I was on the road to perfect health, but it wasn't the case.

I continued with the liver cleanses throughout the spring. During the second one, I got 400 stones out, and during the third, I got 250 out. I was making good progress towards getting two thousand stones out, but the promised improvements were not materializing. In fact, my digestion seemed to be deteriorating.

The flourless chocolate cake was just the start of it. I had gone to one of the very few local restaurants in our new country village, and ordered the only gluten free dish on the menu: steak. I wasn't a big red meat eater.

My girlfriend was vegetarian, so I had never learned how to cook it. The day after, my hemorrhoid bled and bled. I had already given up chocolate after the Seder. Now I gave up red meat too. I mentally crossed that restaurant off my very short list of dining options.

I restricted my diet more, easing up on my sugar consumption and focusing on healthy whole foods, but my energy and enthusiasm for life waned. I became fretful, and could burst into tears at the drop of a hat. I thought it was related to having moved house. It made sense. The initial excitement of moving was over, now I just faced the drudgery of getting the house and garden in order, and the twin daunting tasks of coming up with new friends and a new job. It was understandable that I missed my old life in the city.

To cheer myself up, the next time I went into the city for therapy, instead of just loading up on gluten free staples at upstairs Fairway and going home, I arranged to meet up with my girlfriend for lunch. I'd read online that a Chinese restaurant called Gourmetland had announced the launch of its new gluten free menu. We were going to go check it out.

When we got there, we saw that we were the only customers in the place. The waiter took his time, happy to guide me through my gluten free options, and even told me about some gluten free specials that weren't on the menu. I was happy to hear that I could order gluten free fried rice. It was one of my favorite dishes and I hadn't had it since I'd gone gluten free.

Our dishes were brought to the table and we started to eat. After a minute, we noticed the white-coated chef emerging from the kitchen, beckoning to our waiter, and engaging him in an intense discussion in the corner. Every now and then, he gestured towards our table. We couldn't understand a word of their exchange, but it was obvious that we were the topic of their heated discussion.

Eventually, the red-faced waiter approached our table.

"I'm very very sorry," he said, removing my dish of fried rice. "But we made a mistake. There are two versions of our fried rice, and the chef made the one that is not gluten free. He'll make you another one right away."

My girlfriend and I looked at each other, appalled. I felt the contaminated food clench like a rock in my stomach.

"No, thank you," I said. "I don't want any more."

"I'll make sure it's gluten free," the waiter said. "I'm so sorry."

"I'm done," I said.

"Me too," said my girlfriend, and the hand-wringing waiter apologized to us all the way out the door.

Nothing happened that evening. I made my way home and ate my dinner, feeling fine. But I knew that this was my pattern. In the early days when I still made mistakes and gotten glutened, I never felt bad right away, it always started the next morning. This time it began in the middle of the night.

I woke up to find that my left arm had gone numb, as if I'd been lying on it and it had lost circulation. I rolled over in an attempt to free it up, but realized that it had been free all along. It had gone numb for no reason.

In the morning it was my feet that lost sensation. They went through cycles of numbness and tingling. And then my mouth and my scalp joined in on the action. This was all in addition to an intense version of my usual gluten headache, which had come with the extra twist of an odd kind of tunnel vision. Everything looked a shade darker than usual, with shadows around the periphery. All in all, it was a miserable day, because of the symptoms I was suffering through, and also because of what they signified.

It was a slap in the face. I wasn't as supremely healthy as I'd thought. I had blithely been going along, thinking that I would feel better and better as long as I stuck to the gluten free diet. After the first few weeks, I'd even stopped reading the discussion forums on celiac.com, thinking I had it all figured out. But it was obvious now that I needed to do some research. I was just four months into this thing, and clouds had already gathered on the horizon. I needed to know what they meant.

I went online and studied the celiac forums. I read some posts written by people who had the numbness and tingling I was experiencing. Apparently the medical term for it was 'neuropathy' and some people with celiac disease had neuropathy as their main symptom instead of the more common diarrhea and gastrointestinal symptoms.

One woman said:

"The numbness is getting worse. My doctor says there is nothing he can give me for it. The only treatment is to stay strictly on the gluten free diet. I am doing my best, and hope and pray that this will stop it from progressing."

This sounded serious. Most people on the forums talked about how their gluten symptoms got a lot more frightening the longer they stayed on the gluten free diet. Suddenly, I was scared. It looked like there was no margin for error.

◈◈

And then, out of the blue, I got a yeast infection. I didn't know what it was, because I'd never had one before, but my girlfriend explained that this was what my vaginal itching and discomfort was. She told me that a very effective natural remedy was to take a clove of garlic, nick it with a knife, and use it as a vaginal suppository. I tried this, and it worked. For a little while.

The yeast infection came back the next week, and along with it came the incredible and overwhelming certainty that I was Doomed. I could do nothing except sob hysterically until the feeling passed. It didn't go away entirely. I walked around from then on feeling that I was a little bit doomed, but I was able to not actively wail about it.

I brought this symptom and emotional reaction in to my therapist at my next session. I almost felt embarrassed at how obvious this was, what an easy pitch I was lobbing into her lap. These were the kinds of sessions therapists waited for, right?

"What do you think your body is trying to tell you?" she asked gently.

I shook my head mutely.

"How do you feel?" she asked.

"Like I'm drowning in horror," I said.

"Is there a part of you that holds a memory?" she said. "An event in the past connected with that horror?"

I tried. I searched inside myself, but there was no other part of me holding anything. Just me alone, trapped in a pit of physical and emotional misery.

Talk therapy was not going to fix this. Well, if the problem was not psychological, then it clearly had to be physical. I saw now that I had been playing around with cleansing, doing a little parasite cleanse here, a little liver flushing there. It was clear to me now that I had to get serious with the cleansing. It was time for the big guns.

I took out a video that Margaret had lent me. It was an interview with the natural healer Dr. Richard Schulze. He was famous for his 'Incurables Program,' and in the video, he listed all the cleanses that made up the complete program. He talked about how powerful it was to cleanse the liver, kidneys, lungs, all systems of the body at once. But he emphasized that none of it would have any effect if the most important cleanse was omitted.

This of course was the bowel cleanse. If the bowel was congested with gunk, if it was backed up and leaking toxins into the bloodstream, none of the other cleanses would make the slightest difference. In fact, they would probably make things worse. The bowel was the channel through which toxins exited the body, and it had to be clear before any healing could happen.

I saw now that I had been doing everything backwards. I should have done the bowel cleanse first. A congested bowel was clearly the root of all my problems. Diseased conditions in my bowel had brought on an overgrowth of candida, and caused those crazy yeast infections. An inflamed bowel had caused my hemorrhoid to flare up, and had made my reaction to gluten frighteningly intense. Maybe it had even caused my whole case of gluten intolerance.

Well, I was going to get started right away and fix this whole mess. I was going to cleanse my bowel until all my ills were cured.

I went online, ordered the tinctures and powders I

needed, and over the next two months, mixed up and choked back a special bowel cleansing drink three times a day. It was jet black in color because it contained powdered charcoal, which was excellent at absorbing toxins from the intestines. But that wasn't all it contained. There were six other ingredients, each with its own healing and cleansing properties, from apple pectin powder which would sweep the gunk out of my intestines, to slippery elm which would soothe and heal my inner tissues.

On top of all this, I was also running a simultaneous parasite cleanse because I knew for sure I had parasites, and was on a sugar-free-whole-food-anti-candida diet which I sometimes interspersed with periods of juicing and raw food fasts. I was doing healing enemas twice a week, and was also taking milk thistle every day, just in case my problems were due to congestion in my liver. It was a pretty hard core healing regimen, a kind of lite version of the incurables program. It wasn't a million miles from the cleanse Margaret had used to cure her cancer.

The result?

I felt worse. Much much worse. Physically, I had started to have unexplained episodes of weakness and stomach pain at 11am every morning. If I ate foods that contained a lot of potassium like potatoes or bananas, I felt lightheaded, like I might pass out. Despite the fact that I was on a healing bowel cleanse and took frequent enemas, my hemorrhoid bled regularly. My physical strength and stamina were ebbing away. I was spending more and more days resting in bed.

And how was I doing mentally? Frankly, I was turning into a basket case. I was moody and irritable much of the time. When my girlfriend was around, I couldn't help picking on her and starting stupid fights. When she wasn't, I resented being left alone. After a few short weeks of reprieve during the first phase of the parasite cleanse, the hysterical yeast infections returned. It seemed that every day, I was fighting some kind of inner demon. One night, I developed an irrational fear of the light and shadow playing against my bedroom wall. It was just headlights from the parking lot across the street, casting strange shadows through the trees and brush, but my mind interpreted it as a mysterious and sinister invasion of my space. I stood outside my bedroom window in the dark, trying to catch whatever it was, but it got away.

I lay in bed for hours, staring at the ceiling, wondering what could be chewing up my insides. It had to be something huge. Only a seriously scary disease could stand up against all of the cleansing firepower I was throwing at it. When pain lingered on the left side of my body, I imagined that I had a tumor in my pancreas. Those were very aggressive. I'd probably be dead in a month. On days when my thoughts and emotions were particularly haywire, I pictured a tumor eating up my brain. The worst of it was that I was completely aware of how nutty I was.

A part of me could tell very clearly that I was losing it. But nothing I told myself, nothing I did, nothing I ate or didn't eat, nothing I took could make it stop.

I knew that I was out of my depth, so I reached out to my girlfriend, trying to explain to her that there was something wrong.

"I have a weird feeling that I might be dying," I said.

"What do you mean?" she asked. "Dying of what?"

"I don't know," I said.

"Is there something wrong? Do you feel sick?" she asked.

"Well, I had those yeast infections," I said. "And I…"

I couldn't put it into words that made sense. What could I say? I have a terrifying incurable disease that might just be moodiness?

"…I don't feel right," I finished lamely.

"Did you maybe eat some gluten?" she asked.

No I didn't, I thought. But I didn't have enough energy to contradict her. Not enough to open my mouth and also keep the tears at bay. Wasn't I saying it right? Couldn't she hear that I was asking for help?

"You've been doing great," she said. "This is just a temporary setback. You'll figure it out. You always do."

I nodded and left the room. I could understand why she wasn't interested. I always had some kind of health project going on. Why should she get drawn into this one? Her message was clear. Go away and figure this out on your own.

On a day when the yeast was up and active, I was sitting in my therapist's office, trying to explain to her what was happening to me.

"I feel like I'm decomposing," I said. "It's inside me. In my gut. It's eating me from the inside out."

"I see," she said. "And on what other level can we ask the question, *What's inside my gut?*"

"No other level!" I exploded. "This is physical! This is happening to me today! This is not a memory!"

I felt like I was dying by inches in front of everybody's eyes, and nobody saw or cared. And yet, if I was really dying, why wasn't it obvious what I was dying of? What were my terrible symptoms? Why wasn't I rushing to a doctor for help?

Ha! Because I could imagine how that conversation would go.

"I have a number of problems that all have been increasing in severity in the past few months. I wonder if there's some underlying connection between them all."

"Okay, well, what are your problems?"

"Constipation—"

"Here's a laxative."

"Hemorrhoids—"

"Here are some suppositories."

"Yeast infections—"

"Here's some Monistat."

"And a growing sense of Doom."

"Would you like Prozac or Paxil for that?"

Why pay $200 to have that idiotic conversation. There was no point in going to a doctor until I knew what was wrong with me, and despite all of my efforts, I still didn't know.

∽⑬∾

Fall was approaching. It was now nine months since I'd had my last amalgam filling removed, and five months since the beginning of my mysterious spiral into ill health. I'd done some work on the garden, planted and harvested, even done some canning, but I'd made no real progress in my job search. I was spending far too much time at home alone, brooding over my health. The story I told myself and others was that I was working on editing my novel. But most of my time in front of the computer was spent searching the internet, trying to find out what the hell was wrong with me. I had moved well past WebMD at this point. Mainstream medicine did not have the answers. I trawled every natural healing website I could find, plugged my symptoms into google in every combination I could think of, but only came up with the same tired advice: *If you have digestive problems, try the gluten free diet, try a bowel cleanse, try a liver flush. If you have chronic yeast infections, try having your amalgam fillings removed because mercury toxicity can exacerbate yeast.*

Well my amalgam fillings had been removed long before my yeast got exacerbated. Mercury was the only thing I could definitely cross off my list of suspects. It had left the building months ago. I tried more google searches, but kept coming up with the same frustrating answers. It was all totally useless.

I needed to get out of the house. But I had come to a point where I was pretty sure I couldn't hold down a real job. My thoughts were often clouded with irrational fear. Was I even capable of having normal interactions with normal people? I'd spent so much of the summer alone, I didn't even know. I decided to ease gently back into the workforce.

There was a school for emotionally disturbed kids halfway between the city and our house. They were looking for volunteers to help run their campus farm program. I made an appointment for an interview with the farm director.

Even though I had use of the car every day, I was glad to see that I could take the train and then a local bus to the school. I had become more and more anxious whenever I had to drive. It was as if my brain took too long to comprehend what was coming up in the road in front of me. I had far too many moments looking out the windshield, wondering, What am I looking at? Is that gray thing the road? Or is it a wall? When is the answer going to come to me? Please tell me that I'm not supposed to guess?

As a result, I drove like a scared old lady, which infuriated the drivers behind me on our country two-lane roads, and made me hate driving even more. I only took the car out when I had no other option.

The farm director was very happy to give me the tour of the facilities. It was very impressive. There was a horse riding program, domestic animals like pigs, goats and sheep, as well as exotic creatures like llamas, emus, and birds of prey. As we walked, he asked me about myself, and I fed him the line I'd rehearsed about being a writer working from home who wanted to get out of the house and do some physical work.

"I used to work as a nanny when I lived in the city," I said. "I did that part time, and then wrote the rest of the time."

"That's great," he said.

We paused and leaned on a fence, watching an intern shoveling horse manure into a wheelbarrow.

"I'm afraid it's not very glamorous work," he said. "A lot of shoveling, a lot of cleaning out stalls. But I'm sure we can work in some time where you can assist with classes and have more interaction with the children."

I nodded and smiled, but secretly planned to avoid any situation where I was expected to act like a real grown-up. I was scared that I wouldn't be able to perform, that my brain would spaz out, and I'd be unmasked as being just as emotionally disturbed as the kids I was supposed to take care of.

And so one day a week, I got on the train and took the bus to the school and worked like a dog doing the most menial chores I could find. It was work that drained my already-depleted energy stores, but I was glad to do it because it made me feel somewhat like a productive member of society. Once every other week, I got on the train and went into the city to see my therapist. And the rest of the time, I spent at home, tinkering with my cleanses, trying very hard not to fight with my girlfriend when she was around, and trying very hard to solve my health mystery when she was not.

In my recent reading on the internet, everything seemed to circle back to mercury. Everywhere I looked, the answer was mercury. It was so frustrating. How could mercury possibly be the culprit in my case? The last trace of amalgam had been removed from my mouth nine months before. Mercury hadn't made me particularly sick during amalgam removal, a time when my exposure to it was at its highest. Why would it make me sick now, when the last traces of it should be fading away?

But with all the talk online about the connection between yeast infections and mercury, I was forced to open my mind to the idea.

For mercury to make me sick now, there would have to be some problem with the way my body was getting rid of it. How did the human body excrete mercury anyway?

I looked it up, and found that mercury came out through sweat, urine, and was also exported from the liver via bile, and traveled through the colon to be excreted as feces. I could feel that something was wrong with my digestive system. Was mercury doing it? Was that because the mercury was coming out too fast? Or maybe it was coming out too slow? Was it building up in my gut and causing problems? Should I quit the bowel cleanse to slow things down? Or redouble my efforts to speed things up? I truly had no idea.

I decided to hedge my bets by dropping the harsher ingredients of the bowel cleanse like bentonite clay and sticking with the soothing ones like aloe vera and peppermint. Of course this didn't fix anything. The days and weeks passed, and I sank deeper and deeper into the mercury pit.

There was nobody around me who could help. Even worse, I was losing faith in my ability to help myself. The invisible force I was grappling with was bigger than me, and I didn't know how long I could keep up the fight. Irrational thoughts and dark feelings took over my head for hours at a time, while in a tiny corner, I held my ground and told myself that it wasn't real, that it would pass and I would soon feel like myself again. But as time went by, I felt like there was less of 'me' and more of 'it.' Whatever it was that was chewing up my body and soul was gaining ground.

I tried to communicate what I was experiencing to my therapist. By that point, it had gotten harder to talk. The part of me that could translate my feelings into words seemed like it was eaten up already. But she had a long history of sitting with me, listening patiently, waiting while I found words for the indescribable.

"Are you feeling fear?" she asked.

I paused and considered.

"Yes," I said.

"Can you describe it?"

"It's a fear of the thing that's happening to me," I said, groping for the right words. "I'm afraid because there's something coming to get me that's going to destroy me."

"Who is it?" she asked. "Is there a face?"

"No," I said. "It's not a person."

"What is it?"

"Just...destruction," I said. "This thing that's going to run though me and tear me apart."

"Is it violent?"

"No," I said. "It's invisible, it's quiet."

"Why does it want to destroy you?"

"I don't think it *wants* anything," I said. "This is just what it does. It'll take me over and I won't be able to stop it."

"And then what?"

"I'll lose," I said. "My feelings won't be my real feelings anymore, just torn-up crap. I won't be me. I'll be not-me. The real me will be gone."

I took a deep breath. Tears began to leak out of my eyes.

"It's getting closer," I said. "I feel like I'm standing at the edge of a void. It's going to reach up and swallow me."

She nodded, and took a deep breath.

"This sounds like an existential issue," she said. "Getting trapped all alone in a vacuum of meaninglessness."

I nodded. This sounded right.

"Like there's nothing good out there," she said. "No feeling that you'll be taken care of. Just isolation."

"Yeah."

"This kind of stuff can come up around spiritual issues," she said. "I know you grew up Catholic. Do you believe in God?"

"No," I said.

"Nothing? No Higher Power, no life after death?"

"Nope."

"And when did that shift occur?" she asked.

I could tell right away that she was way off the mark. Nothing that was happening inside me was connected to my lack of belief in God. But since I'd paid for the hour, I talked for a while about religion. It was good to feel the back and forth of a normal conversation, even if it did nothing to shed light on my issues. It helped a little just to talk about it, to have someone hear what I was going through.

At the end of the session, she checked in.

"So what's coming up for you this week?" she asked.

"My birthday." Birthdays had always been hard for me, and she knew it. They always dropped me into a space of childhood disappointment.

"How old are you going to be?"

"Thirty three," I said. "The same age as Jesus when he died."

She rolled her eyes. "Did you have to go there?"

"No, I didn't," I said. "But if you don't laugh, you cry, right?"

After my session, I went downtown to the Russian Baths on 10th street. I'd been there before with Margaret when she was in the midst of her cleanse. I hoped that sweating the mercury out would make me feel better. And it did, for a day or so, but then the darkness crowded in again.

On my birthday, I cancelled plans to go have dinner in the city with my girlfriend and spent the day in bed, taking stock. What a terrible year it had been. It had started out well with amalgam removal and getting on the gluten free diet, but then everything had gone to hell in a hand basket. All the parasite formula, liver flushes, months of bowel cleansing, aloe vera, sweating, therapy, what did I have to show for it? I was worse off than before I'd done any of it.

I feel defeated, I wrote in my diary. *I'm out of ideas.*

I had to accept the fact that it was time to give up. No more wasting my time doing internet research. No more learning about bowel cleansing herbs or healing enemas. It was time to stop. I wasn't able to fix this, and the best thing I could do was admit I was powerless and quit struggling.

It felt good to let go. A quiet peace came over me. I could stop running around like a rat in a maze, encountering the same dead ends over and over again.

The next time I took out my computer, I didn't reach for the same google searches. No more typing in 'heavy metal candida' or 'mercury bowel cleanse.' That exercise in futility was over. I'd put so much energy into it, and at the end of it all, I still didn't even know if mercury was really my problem. It was just a blind guess. All I'd done was spend months stumbling around on the internet, picking up random ideas.

I didn't regret trying the cleansing. It had cured Margaret, she was someone I knew, I'd watched her go through the process. But mercury poisoning? That was just an abstract idea I'd latched onto. I'd never met anyone who'd had it. I didn't have the first clue what it looked like, or how a person could even tell if they really had it.

I paused for a moment, thinking about that idea. How would a person go about finding out for sure if they had mercury poisoning? Wouldn't it help if they met someone else who had exactly the same problems they had? Someone who had their fillings out, and then turned into a yeast-filled basket case? Wouldn't that be very revealing?

What if I could find someone who was struggling in the exact same way that I was struggling? Someone who was willing to tell the truth about what was going on inside them? Wouldn't it say so much? Far more than a hundred half-baked internet bullshit articles about mercury and candida ever could?

I brought up google, and my fingers hovered over the keyboard. How exactly could I find a real live mercury toxic person who was willing to tell the actual truth about their life?

I typed in 'mercury stories' and hit search.

Bingo.

In the first story, a 34-year-old man talked about how he had increasing depression, fatigue, and a host of mysterious little ailments: *I attributed it all to hypoglycemia and possibly aging. I ate myself into hypoglycemia in my younger years with an unbelievably horrible diet. "Now I'm paying for it," I thought.*

I nodded at the screen. Hypoglycemia and turning into a little old lady. That's how I'd explained everything for a while too.

But for this man, hypoglycemia didn't explain everything anymore because he went on to develop chronic yeast infections and very serious depression.

Reading this, I got goose bumps on my arms. It was true, then. Yeast and mercury were connected. I inhaled the rest of his story, and a cog began to turn in my brain when he said that his hypoglycemia disappeared in the weeks following amalgam removal. My hypoglycemia had disappeared in the weeks following amalgam removal too.

In the next mercury story I read, a woman talked about yeast problems too. And I really sat up and paid attention when she talked about getting a mysterious swelling in her salivary glands similar to the episode of the mumps I'd gotten out of the blue when I first got sick. She also had large boils that burst and wept pus. I'd had one of them when I was in college, I'd even had surgery done on it to make sure it healed properly.

The next person mentioned yeast too, and then described going on a gluten free diet. The next talked about gluten intolerance and also about having abnormally cold hands and feet, something that my girlfriend frequently pointed out I suffered from. Others talked about their hair falling out. Mine had been falling out since my college days, I had to keep it short to make sure I didn't kill the bathroom drain wherever I lived.

There was talk of lots of symptoms I didn't have, like hives, excruciating facial pain, or memory loss. But the hits kept coming. More than one person mentioned chronic constipation. Most everyone talked about the vicious depression, and the feeling that you were aging before your time. My mind pinged with recognition over and over again. I was just like these people, going through so many things that they were going through.

The cog in my brain that had started to turn when I read the first story suddenly engaged with the big wheels in my mind, and something that I'd believed for the past year got turned on its head.

What if it wasn't the gluten? Those first marvelous months after I'd seen the dentist, that miraculous improvement? What if it had solely been caused by amalgam removal?

I'd been operating under the impression that getting on the gluten free diet had made everything better. But what if that simply wasn't true? What if something much deeper had been going on?

My mind ran through everything that had happened to me, all the way back to that first conversation about gluten with the dentist.

Duh. Of course. The dentist! She'd told me to go gluten free. It wasn't some side issue, some random coincidence. She was mercury toxic too! She'd probably sucked up more mercury in her career than anyone I'd ever met.

My mind buzzed as the facts rearranged themselves into their true order. I'd been wrong all along. I'd thought that celiac, yeast and all my other food intolerances all sprang from the same diseased origin, my congested bowel. I could see that I was right on one level. These problems certainly were connected. But my bowel was just another innocent bystander.

It was mercury who was behind all this.

Mercury had caused my gluten intolerance. Mercury had given me yeast. I was losing my mind because of mercury, and my hemorrhoid was bleeding because of mercury.

I couldn't prove it, but I had a strong feeling that

every single health problem I'd had since the age of 16 had mercury's fingerprints all over it.

I finally understood why things had gone so wrong for me, but it still wasn't clear how to put them right. One of the stories described getting chelation therapy that involved DMPS injections. The guy talked about them as if they were a positive experience, but the side effects sounded brutal. I was going to steer well clear of that treatment. But what else could I try?

The website I was on highly recommended two books on mercury poisoning: *It's All in Your Head* by Hal Huggins and *Amalgam Illness* by Andrew Hall Cutler. I ordered both books immediately. In the meantime, I got on the Yahoo group devoted to discussing the Cutler book so I could learn more.

I could feel a knot of fear I'd been carrying inside me for months gradually dissolve. Finally, finally I had found out what was wrong. Armed with the right information, I could do whatever needed to be done to fix it all up in no time.

I heaved a sigh of relief. Any minute now it would all be over, and I'd finally get my life back.

III

❧❧

DMSA

Amalgam Illness arrived in the mail. I read it cover to cover in two days. It confirmed everything I'd suspected. Mercury was at the root of it all. It was a sneaky, broad-ranging toxin that attacked almost every system in the body. Fixing this was not going to be a simple matter. It had taken years for things to go wrong, it wasn't just a case of waving a magic wand and everything would be made right. I cursed the day that I sat in Dr. Whelan's chair and gave the wrong answer to the question: *Silver or white?* The more I read, the more information I absorbed, the angrier I got. Mitochondria? I didn't even know they existed. They were supposed to fill my cells with energy? And mercury was screwing that up? Great. Fucking awesome.

Amalgam Illness was full of advice on how to treat mercury poisoning, it laid out a whole plan of action. The first step was to get on some supplements. The whole second half of the book was basically a long list of vitamins, herbs and minerals that could knock mercury symptoms on the head. As I turned the pages, I made a list of the ones that might help my particular problems.

Some of these supplements I was currently taking, like milk thistle. Others were old friends like ginkgo biloba and chromium. I had known that they had helped me in the past. Why on Earth had I stopped taking them? It was all vanity. I had enjoyed the image of being a healthy person, someone who didn't need that kind of support. So stupid.

Well vanity was out the window now. I pulled out all my supplement bottles, lined them up on the counter, and drove to the drugstore to buy an old-lady pill minder to keep track of them all.

These supplements were:

Magnesium

Milk Thistle

Flax Oil Capsules

Vitamin C

Zinc

Ginkgo Biloba

Glutamine

Chromium

Probiotics

Then I ordered some more likely candidates online:

Vitamin E

CoQ10

Forskolin

Digestive enzymes with ox bile

B3 as Niacinamide

I also ordered the two over-the-counter chelators discussed in *Amalgam Illness*—Alpha Lipoic Acid and DMSA. When they arrived, I put them to one side. I wasn't at all sure that I would ever use them. Chelators were powerful drugs that were chemically structured to enter the body, stir up mercury, grab onto little atoms of it, and usher it out of the body via urine or feces. The more I read about their effects on other people on the Frequent Dose Chelation Yahoo Group, the surer I became that these drugs would cause overwhelmingly nasty side effects if I ever took them. Still, I wanted to have them around just in case.

When the supplements arrived in the mail, I opened up the bottles and tried to jam them into the already-packed compartments of the old-lady pill minder. They wouldn't fit. I had to drive back to the drugstore and upgrade to the jumbo size.

The first regular-sized pill holder ended up housing my breakfast supplements, and the jumbo took care of the dinner supplements, which were much greater in number because they included eight flax oil capsules. The few stray extras that went with lunch or at bedtime, I took straight out of the bottle. And every day I still drank a little aloe vera juice with a drop of peppermint oil, a pinch of slippery elm and a squirt of cayenne tincture. These were what I identified as the 'gentle' elements of the bowel cleanse I had been on. I didn't want to stop taking them because I felt that they were doing something good for my colon. My new regimen made me think of a fragment of a poem I'd read when I was young:

Every day for their ills
They take dozens of pills
So they rattle like mad when they run

I hoped that these dozens of pills were going to have some kind of positive effect.

I could definitely feel the supplements making a difference. My mood got a bit lighter. But since I was so far in the hole, 'a bit lighter' was still far from okay. And unsurprisingly, within days, I started having some side effects. Niacinamide didn't sit well with me, which was predictable as I'd reacted badly to taking B complex in the past. CoQ10 made me feel good in the couple of hours after I took it, but it also made my heart pound in an alarming way, even if I was sitting doing nothing. I tried a lower dose but the same thing happened, so I stopped taking it. Forskolin seemed to be bringing me back to my old hypoglycemic days, so I quit that too. Back on zinc, the nausea reminded me why I'd stopped taking it in the first place. Cutler stressed how important it was for mercury toxic people to address their zinc deficiency, so I did my best to take a tiny nibble of the chewable whenever I could stand it.

The digestive enzymes were hard to judge. They seemed to make my stomach burn a little bit when I took them. I tried only taking them with meals that were heavy in protein, and that seemed to help. Were they making a difference in how I felt? The jury was out.

I settled into my new regimen, and after a week or two, the day dawned when I thought, Well, this is as good as things are going to get if I only use supplements.

It wasn't anywhere near good enough.

❧

That wasn't a big surprise, given what I was going through. I learned from *Amalgam Illness* that my body was in the throes of a viciously powerful mercury detox reaction. People on the forums affectionately referred to it as 'The Dump Phase.' During my many years of exposure to amalgam, my cells and organs had slowly gotten filled up with mercury. But after those amalgams got removed, there was no more mercury coming in. My falling mercury levels had made me feel great in the weeks after amalgam removal.

But once my bloodstream got clear enough, the automatic detox began. The dam burst, and all the mercury stored up in my cells started pouring out. What had trickled in slowly over a period of 16 years, was now gushing out in a period of 16 months. My kidneys and liver couldn't excrete the stuff fast enough. I was drowning in mercury, and there wasn't a thing I could do about it.

That wasn't technically true. There was something I could do about it, but I was afraid to take that step. The next logical thing for me to try was chelation.

The chelation protocol described in *Amalgam Illness* didn't involve any scary injections or IVs. It wasn't meant to invoke an unbearable healing crisis. On the contrary, the protocol was designed to remove mercury from the body as carefully and gently as possible. I read this and I tried to believe it, but I still doubted it. How could it be gentle enough for me? My body couldn't tolerate chocolate. If meat made me bleed, how on earth could I withstand the side effects of mercury-mobilizing drugs?

I needed to talk through my options, but I couldn't bring this to my girlfriend. Life with her over the past month had been one continuous rolling ongoing fight. When we spoke, I did my best to be reasonable, but it was like I was possessed, like a mercury demon was using me as a mouthpiece. Every conversation devolved into conflict. I believed that she still loved me, but I was also pretty sure at this point that she didn't particularly like me.

So I took it to my therapist.

"Okay," I began. "It turns out that I've been poisoned."

"I see," she said. "You feel poisoned."

"No!" I said. "Work with me here! I have been literally poisoned. In the real world. Not in some metaphorical way. By mercury."

It was hopeless. There was so much to explain. *Your dentist shouldn't have given you chlorella. What is chlorella?*

The whole hour was up before I'd even gotten anywhere near the burning question. Should I do this? Should I take DMSA? What if it did terrible things to me?

When I got home, I got online and searched the Frequent Dose Chelation forum for mentions of starting DMSA. *It made my gums bleed*, someone said. That was worrying. Would my bleeding hemorrhoid get out of control like it had during amalgam removal? Then someone else said, *It acted like an antidepressant for me. Thank God for DMSA.*

A tiny fire of hope ignited inside me. I ran a search for 'DMSA antidepressant' and it popped up all over. What if it did that for me too?

⋞⋟

So a few days later, I embarked on my first round of chelation with DMSA. A 'round' in the Frequent Dose Chelation protocol meant taking DMSA at regular four-hour intervals around the clock for three days without stopping. This included waking up at night to take doses. I gathered up all the clocks and watches in the house that had alarms, and decided that a noon-4pm-8pm-midnight-4am-8am schedule would be the easiest to keep track of with its multiples of the number 4. I set three alarm clocks for the nighttime doses, and decided the kitchen timer would do for the daytime.

Cutler recommended 50 to 100mg of DMSA per dose. The four hour timing interval was set in stone, but doses were flexible. I decided to try 12.5mg. I figured I could handle a quarter of what the average person could take, and besides, it was exactly half of a 25mg capsule.

Splitting the contents of a capsule in half was no joke, especially the teeny ones that DMSA came in. It wasn't just a case of getting the capsule and dumping half of it down the sink. DMSA was pricey, thirty dollars a bottle. I couldn't throw half of it out. I had some empty capsules that I'd bought at the health food store, large ones it was easy to pour powder into. So I dumped the contents of the tiny DMSA capsule onto a piece of paper, used a knife to divide the pile in half, then carefully brushed each pile onto a folded post-it note to pour it into the large empty capsules. It was a tricky, painstaking process. I got tired of it after making up half a dozen doses, enough to cover one day. Side effects would probably halt this whole process by then, anyway. I decided not to make up any more.

I took my first dose at noon, and waited to see what would happen. It was pretty subtle, but over the next hour, I could feel the dose taking hold. It wasn't anything bad, I just felt a little spaced out. I could feel it winding down after three hours, and then ramping up again after I took my dose at 4pm. It really wasn't a big deal.

My 8pm dose was fine, but one of the alarms didn't go off at midnight, and I was late taking the dose. It was okay to take it when I actually woke up at 12:17am, because it wasn't more than an hour late. Otherwise, I would have had to stop the round. I wasn't sure what had woken me. I had been in the middle of a vivid dream where my head was below my shoulders, all of my body parts were rearranged.

I woke on time at 4am, taking my dose by the light of a flashlight, so as not to disturb my girlfriend. I fell back into an endless night of dreams that felt so real, it was almost like I was awake while I was dreaming.

My second day on round I was supposed to work at the school farm program. Getting up in the morning wasn't a problem. I had decided the night before that I would call in sick if I needed to, but as far as I could tell, I felt perfectly fine. My 8am dose didn't even seem to have a great effect on me, so instead of going to the bother of splitting more capsules, I decided to go ahead and try 25mg for my second day of chelation.

I wasn't going to carry my kitchen timer around with me at work, so I set noon and 4pm alarms on my digital watch. I was helping one of the interns, clearing out stalls when our work was interrupted by the alarm on my watch sounding at noon.

"Time for lunch," I announced, immediately downing tools and heading for the lunchroom, where my bottle of pills sat in my coat pocket. I didn't want to get sidetracked and forget to take my dose.

The school day happened to end at 4pm, just in time for my next dose, and I wound up working with the same intern when my alarm went off again.

"I guess it's quitting time," I said, hastily putting away my tools and going to fetch my coat.

"You set an alarm for that?" she called after me.

I turned around and shrugged. "I guess."

On my way home from work, I looked back over my day. I had assisted with horse riding classes, cleaned out stalls, carried buckets of feed all over the place. Just like every Tuesday, I'd been on my feet all day, working like a dog. But unlike other Tuesdays, coming home on the train, I wasn't slumped with exhaustion. I wasn't pining for my couch, where I could sit and stuff my face to feed my bottomless hunger until I collapsed into bed. This Tuesday, I felt as fresh at the end of the day as I did at the beginning. I began to entertain the thought that something good was happening.

On the third day of the round, I doubled my dose again to 50mg, since 25mg had gone so well. I went out and did my shopping, coming up with good ideas for sewing projects when I visited the local craft store. The day was perfectly pleasant, except I had a slight headache throughout the day, and my gums felt a little tender, just as expected. I took my last dose at 4pm, and at 8 o'clock, when it was all wearing off and winding down, I was in the kitchen, talking to my girlfriend as we prepared dinner.

We were having a good couple of days, and I felt that it was time to open up to her a little about my recent discoveries. I was explaining chelation to her while she chopped broccoli and I got out the tomato sauce. As I talked, I began to feel kind of stoned.

"How long do you chelate for?" she asked.

"People usually do three days on and four days off," I said.

"No," she said. "I mean, how many weeks do you do the rounds for before you get better?"

"Not weeks," I said. "Months. It's going to be months before my dump phase is over. I'm pretty sure it's going to take another six months. Maybe more."

"And you'll be better then?" she asked. "When? Late next spring? Early summer?"

"It depends," I said.

Cutler talked a lot in *Amalgam Illness* about the mercury stored in the brain. It didn't pour out during the dump phase, it was trapped behind the blood-brain barrier. Brain mercury was actually the cause of a lot of 'body' symptoms, because the brain was the control center for so many of the body's processes. The only way to fix those mercury symptoms was to do weekly rounds with a different chelator called ALA.

"What does it depend on?" she asked.

"How much mercury made it into my brain while I had amalgams," I said. "There's no way to test it. But that's the big measure of how bad it is. My case of broccoli poisoning—"

She laughed.

"I mean, mercury poisoning," I said.

I stood in the middle of the kitchen and looked around scratching my head.

"Where did I put the sauce?" I asked, bewildered.

My girlfriend found the full jar, sitting in the sink with the lid off. She took me by the hand and led me to a stool.

"You sit here, and I'll finish the cooking," she said.

I sat and watched her cook, and enjoyed the stoned feeling that rolled over me. By the time an hour had passed, it had faded, and that was the end of my first round of chelation.

I went on the Frequent Dose Chelation board to write a report on how it went. When I checked back the next day, I found some cheerful but alarmed responses from five different people:

"I would stick with a fairly low dose for several rounds before increasing. Better safe than sorry."

"You should not be increasing your dose within a round! You can only increase the dose when you start a new round. Please be careful."

I had no idea that I had been going too fast, or doing something that wasn't recommended. The book said that 50 to 100mg was the recommended dose. I later found out that the Frequent Dose Chelation Yahoo group recommendations were to start very low, at 12.5mg like I had, and not increase your dose until you'd completed three rounds. I felt a bit sheepish that I had been caught doing it wrong, but far more than that, I was glad that these people were watching out for me.

I'd read that there were after-effects, called 'redistribution,' that surfaced in the 24 to 48 hours after a round ended, so I watched to see what would happen. My hemorrhoid started bleeding the day after the round ended, for the first time in a while. But for the next few days, everything was good.

And then, the following week, I began to feel terrible again. Technically, I could have started another round of DMSA. I had done a three-day round, and the required three-day break was over. But my hemorrhoid was still bleeding. I didn't want to make it worse by chelating some more. I stopped taking vitamin C and that slowed the bleeding a bit, but each day, I felt the mercury darkness crowding in on me. Everything in my life felt fraught with difficulty. Every thought seemed to lead down the same cul-de-sac of despair. The mercury monster was gaining ground in my head again.

I started my second round, sticking with a consistent 25mg of DMSA this time. An hour after my first dose, all the difficulty and despair lifted. While on round, my hemorrhoid stopped bleeding. Everything was easier, life was manageable. I had calm and loving conversations with my girlfriend. I felt like a normal and reasonable human being.

The side effects on this second round were minimal. My dreams were vivid again, but less so than last time.

I also was less spaced out on this round. I was disappointed that I didn't have the stoned feeling when I came off it at the end, but was glad that my body was getting used to DMSA and its effects.

I couldn't believe how well things were going. It looked like I had found the answer to my problems. It truly felt like magic. All I had to do now was find the best balance between being on round and being off round, and everything would be fine. I'd have a good chance of making it through the dump phase alive.

My next round was short, not because I planned it that way, but because the 4am alarm failed to wake me in the middle of the second night. I took a few days off, and trying to stay ahead of the mercury, got right back on round again.

This time, I planned to do a round that was seven days long. I hadn't heard of anybody chelating continuously with DMSA, but I'd heard of people doing schedules that were a week on round followed by a week off. If my rounds were longer, maybe I'd be able to find my feet during the long days of reprieve. Chelation was great, I wasn't knocking it, but I was beginning to feel like a yo-yo at the end of a string, bouncing up and down as the rounds came and went. And since the redistribution after-effects were caused by mobilized mercury crashing into the body's tissues, it would be healthier to reduce the frequency of them to twice a month rather than every single week.

Redistribution usually hit me 36 hours after I took my last dose. And indeed, 36 hours after I finished the week-long round, I wasn't feeling great. In fact, I was feeling really weird. I'd felt poorly since I'd gotten up that morning. I'd woken from a night of sleep reminiscent of the time the dentist had given me garlic capsules. It had been one long grueling nightmare, where I'd kept thinking I was waking up, but always I ended up in another nasty dream.

When I'd finally woken up for real to go to work at the farm, I'd been eager to leave my bed and enter the real world. But sitting on the bus going to work, things didn't feel as real as they should. I stared out the window, taking slow, deep calming breaths. This didn't seem to help. It crossed my mind that I was going to pass out. I held my hands out in front of me, but I didn't have the usual stiffness and tingling in my limbs that was my big passing-out warning sign.

I looked at the other passengers on the bus, their backs to me, sitting so still. It suddenly became clear to me that they were not real human beings. They were just bodies, without thoughts or emotions. Empty breathing flesh. I stared out the window again.

This was not good. This was mercury. Redistributing. Into my brain. Right here on the bus. Wiping out my ability to recognize humanity. If I screamed or passed out, would the non-humans around me even notice? Was I even on the bus? Had I ever really woken up? Was I still trapped in a dream? Or was I actually on the bus, but dying?

These thoughts ran through my mind, while a calm, rational part of me analyzed them. I probably wasn't dying, but I wasn't well. There was nothing I could do except go home and lie down. I would stay on the bus until it looped around back to the train station. I would go home and go to bed. I would be fine.

And then, mercifully, it passed. The people were people again. It wasn't a dream. I was fine. In fact, I felt so fine, I got off at my stop and did my day of work without a problem. The whole thing had lasted maybe ten minutes. Just a little redistribution event.

But I never did a long round again. In the run up to Christmas, I settled down into a pattern of 3 days on, 4 days off. It turned out that 36 hours after my round ended, I was often on that same bus going to work. I had a couple more 'moments,' but nothing as intense as that first one. I was glad. I didn't want to stop chelating. DMSA was my life preserver, keeping me afloat in the mercury ocean. Keeping my head above water in the slow tsunami of the dump phase.

❧❧

I spent a lot of time studying the graph of the dump phase in *Amalgam Illness*, wondering when the tide would turn, how long my personal bell curve of mercury suffering would last. I knew that the signal that I'd reached the top of the curve would be that my symptoms would decrease in intensity. But as the rounds went by, whenever I wasn't on DMSA, the mercury madness felt like it was gaining ground.

By the time Christmas rolled around, I had completed my 6th round of DMSA. My girlfriend and I were celebrating the holiday alone together, and it wasn't easy coming up with a menu that fit all of my dietary restrictions. At this point, I couldn't tolerate gluten, meat, sugar, caffeine, milk, nuts, bananas, potatoes...the list went on. We settled on mac and cheese made with rice milk and rice pasta, pancakes made from spaghetti squash, and buttered peas.

In honor of my Irish heritage, I handmade Christmas crackers, and stuffed them with crepe paper hats, plastic toys and jokes. I was very pleased with myself when I wrote an original joke based on our cat's name. (Q: What do you call a process in which a cat wakes you up at midnight, 4am and 8am precisely? A: Blackielation.)

I had been off sugar since the summer because of my persistent yeast problems, but the combination of probiotics and the parasite cleanse seemed to have kept the hysterical yeast infections at bay. Still, the tinea versicolor fungal rash was pretty active. It had spread from my chest, and was now appearing on my back, arms and neck too. But it wasn't itchy, didn't bother me and would go away as soon as I got around to buying some jock itch cream to put on it. Given the fact that things were under control, I decided it would be okay to eat a little sugar, just once, for Christmas.

Hearing about my decision, my girlfriend decided to go all out, and bought a box of gluten free angel food cake mix. We didn't own an electric mixer, so on Christmas Eve, we spent a couple of hours taking turns with an egg beater, cranking away until our arms got sore and we had to hand off to the other person. The mix was thoroughly beaten when we were done, and the cake was a sight to behold when it came out of the oven, light and fluffy and beautiful.

Christmas Dinner was lovely. Cake for dessert was even lovelier. It was my first taste of sugar in months. I had been experimenting with stevia, an herbal sweetener, and putting lots of cinnamon and vanilla essence in my baking to make it seem sweeter. But nothing could duplicate the real thing. Sugar was awesome, I could feel it melting in my mouth and making its way into my bloodstream immediately. I could understand why they used to call it 'crack' in the old days.

The next day, I had another little slice of cake, followed by another, and then one for the road. I stopped there, because I knew that I was slipping into territory where I may regret my actions. I asked my girlfriend to take the rest of the cake away, I didn't want to have anything more to do with it.

The following day I felt out of sorts. It didn't feel like mercury, it was a different kind of tired and irritable, and didn't know what to do with myself. I tried to keep busy, run my errands and snap out of it. But by the end of the day, I felt quite a bit worse, and could feel the beginnings of a sore throat. I went to the mirror to see how red it looked, and when I opened my mouth, I saw not just redness but spots! I had strep!

I took to my bed for a week, feeling hideous. My girlfriend had to bring me all my meals because I could barely sit up. I was miserable, and when I had enough energy to think about it, I berated myself for foolishly playing around with sugar. Mercury was notorious for screwing with the immune system. My various yeast and fungal problems were proof of that. And now I'd gone and helped it by spooning a big dose of immune-suppressing sugar into the mix. Stupid!

By New Year's Eve, I wasn't well yet, and our plans to go into the city for the night were scrapped. I was able to sit up for a few hours and play a board game with my girlfriend and watch a DVD, but I wasn't feeling great. It wasn't just the strep. I had postponed my next round of DMSA because I was sick, and the mercury was crowding into my head. I was losing my grip on myself. I decided to start a round right away.

The days after that round were hideous, I had redistribution followed by two days of menstrual cramps. Every round, it seemed brought worse redistribution than the round before. And the mercury madness was creeping back sooner and sooner. My windows of clarity were getting shorter and shorter. And bouncing back and forth between days of sanity and days of mercury madness was eroding my grip on reality. I began to wonder how much more of it I could take. Was this dump phase ever going to peak?

On a good day in the middle of the next round, I sat my girlfriend down.

"I want to apologize," I said. "For how I've been these past few months. The mercury makes me scared, and when I get scared, I try to control everything around me. Including you."

"It's okay," she said. "It's not like I've been on top of my game either. Let's just try to be better, okay?"

I closed my eyes for a second, doing my best to come up with words that would explain what I needed to say.

"That's the thing," I said. "I don't think I can be better. The mercury's not going away as fast as I'd hoped. There's a good chance I'm going to get worse."

"But you're doing your rounds," she protested. "You've figured it out."

I shook my head. "The DMSA isn't keeping up with it," I said. "Things are getting harder."

"What do you mean, 'harder'?" she said.

"Just promise me something," I said. "That you'll take care of things. For us. Make decisions for us. If I tell you

I can't trust my judgment anymore."

"You're sounding a bit crazy right now," she said.

"No," I said. "This is me being sane. This is why I need to tell you this now. Because I may not be able to communicate with you later on."

"Why?" she asked. "Where are you going?"

"I'm not going anywhere," I said. "Please. Please promise me that you'll take care of things. If it looks like I'm not able to."

"Okay, but I don't believe you. I think you're overreacting."

"Promise me," I insisted.

"Okay, okay, I promise."

I heaved a sigh of relief. "Thanks."

The dump phase continued to intensify over the winter. On bad days I clamped down hard and didn't let the mercury demon use me as a mouthpiece. Things got very quiet in our house. It was hard to contain the fear and despair that mercury evoked inside me. It was hard too, to resist the urge to talk things through with my girlfriend. She had always been there for me when I needed her. But I knew that if I began, if I let it out, the mercury demon would inevitably turn the conversation into a hurtful fight. There was nothing real about the thoughts and feelings that came up when the mercury was running high. I did my best to tune out, to ignore whatever jumbled horror was going on in my head.

Ignoring my mercury-induced thoughts and feelings took its toll on my relationship with my girlfriend, but it also eroded my relationship with myself. After a while, it became hard to pick and choose what I was supposed to ignore. I began to automatically suspect the reality of all of my feelings, even the positive ones. I grew distanced from myself, always ready to put up a wall between me and not-me. But still, I couldn't think of any better way of handling what was going on inside me.

My immune system wasn't doing so well either. My body was losing its ability to kill yeast. I joined a candida and yeast forum and began to try out different kinds of natural yeast remedies. Some worked for a little while and then got overpowered, others never worked at all.

I went back to the Frequent Dose Chelation group, looking for answers there. Surely other mercury toxic people had struggled with yeast too. I posted about it, and then went looking through the files section.

Almost immediately I found a document called 'Neutrophils, Yeast and DMSA.' From it, I learned the illuminating fact that DMSA had a tendency to lower neutrophil numbers. And what were neutrophils? They were the white blood cells that were in charge of killing yeast!

Of course! My yeast problems were intensifying not because the dump phase was intensifying, but because

I had been taking so much DMSA. It was killing off my poor neutrophils, and causing the yeast to run wild. When I thought about it, there was no reason for my dump phase to be going on and on like this. In fact, it was probably already over, but this fact was masked by my monstrous case of yeast. My course of action was clear. All I had to do was stop taking DMSA and everything would be fine.

I posted about this on the Frequent Dose Chelation forum. I felt sure that they'd all be blown away by my detective work. Identifying that my dump phase was really over, but masked by a case of yeast? Brilliant!

The moderator of the group replied:

"Andy [Cutler] usually says to keep chelating through the gut problems (and to look for ways to address them). I took an extended break since about last March, when I had a serious infection…the break didn't seem to help anything and I'm counting on chelation to make me feel better."

This took the wind out of my sails. Wasn't it obvious that I was right? Andy's advice sounded way off. Chelating through my yeast problem would involve having to take something big to knock my yeast back, a prescription antifungal. I had no intention of turning up at a doctor's office, asking for help from some idiot who knew less than nothing about mercury. That was the last thing I wanted to do.

It didn't matter anyway. My solution was going to work. All I had to do was stop taking DMSA. My neutrophils would bounce back, the yeast would go away and everything would be fine.

I quit taking DMSA.

Two weeks later, I had totally lost it. Yes, the first week off had been good. The yeast had died down, my color had returned, I'd felt stronger and clearer than I had in a while. But then the mercury horror had reasserted itself. With a vengeance. It was worse than I'd ever experienced before. I was now utterly non-functional. I couldn't make it through the day without getting into bed and sleeping for hours, and I couldn't hold a thought in my head for a second. It had all seemed like a good idea at first, but the smothering cloud of mercury felt unbearable, and as the days went by, it showed no signs of lifting.

I tried to tough it out, but by day 16 off DMSA, I couldn't stand it for one more minute. I caved, and started a round of DMSA. Within an hour, I was feeling better.

I knew now that my dump phase wasn't over. I needed DMSA to get me though. And I knew that I was going to have to get a prescription to take care of the yeast. I looked online, but Diflucan or Nystatin weren't the kinds of things you could buy on eBay. I was going to have to swallow my pride and go to some idiot doctor and ask for help.

I decided to go to the holistic doctor that had his practice next to the local health food store and yoga studio. He'd probably be crackers, but being holistic, there was a chance that he wouldn't write me off automatically as a hypochondriac. I called and made an appointment.

∽§§∾

But before I could go see him, I had to go on vacation. Long before I'd gotten sick, my girlfriend's mother had asked us to accompany her to London. My sister lived in London too, so it all worked out nicely. My girlfriend and I would stay with her, while the older generation hung out at my girlfriend's aunt's.

As I got all my supplements ready for the trip, I realized that I didn't have enough DMSA to complete my next round. I'd been so gung-ho about quitting that I hadn't ordered another bottle when I started running low. I got online and ordered it immediately, hoping that it would arrive before we left on the trip.

It didn't.

I brought along the half-round I had, vaguely thinking that I would grit my teeth for a couple of days, and then start the round right before I left. It would be fine.

It wasn't.

I had been stretching the gap between rounds to minimize DMSA's effect on my yeast. I'd managed to stretch it up to twelve days off before we left on our trip. It looked like I was going to be okay for the first week and a half of the trip. But after fourteen days off, the mercury descended on me with a thump. I expected it to make me tired like it had the time I'd tried to quit DMSA. That would be fine. My sister was cool. I could just lie in bed and chat with her and have the kids play around us on the bed.

But this time, the mercury didn't only make me tired. It also had a profound effect on my brain. It emptied out and I was blank. No words inside me. Normally there was always something going on inside my head, even if it was mercury garbage. Now things had gone eerily quiet.

My girlfriend, picking up that something was wrong, began to follow me around my sister's house. I found an empty room and sat there, relieved to be alone, but a couple of minutes later, my girlfriend appeared and sat beside me. Right beside me! I couldn't stand it! I felt that if she asked me a question, I'd scream.

I got up and left the room and found somewhere quiet, but she followed me all over again. This went on and on. And the eye contact! Excruciating. Why did everyone keep trying to look at me?

As the hours went by, things got stranger inside me. It was clear that I was acting very oddly and I had to explain to my sister and girlfriend what was going on.

"I need to take DMSA, but I don't have enough," I said. "So this is what's happening to me."

My sister wrote down 'DMSA' on a piece of paper and said she'd ask the chemist about it the next day.

"I'm pretty sure it's not the kind of thing they stock at Boots," I said.

I went to bed, hoping that the worst was over.

I was alone when I woke up the next morning, my girlfriend had gone to meet a friend for lunch. I was relieved to be alone, because I felt absolutely desperate. My

confusing. Where was all the medical paraphernalia? Where was the desk? Was the doctor going to just come in and sit in the other armchair and talk to me? That was so unlikely, doctors needed their props. This was probably just another waiting room.

After a few minutes, the door opened and a tall, skinny man with curly hair popped in. I jumped up, ready to follow him to the examining room, but after he shook my hand and introduced himself, he indicated the armchairs and we sat down.

"So," he smiled broadly, "What can I do for you?"

I found the smile disconcerting. I'd never seen a doctor who seemed so happy to meet me before. But I knew my line and I trotted it out.

"I've been having persistent yeast problems," I said. "And I need a prescription for Diflucan."

"Sure, sure," he said. "No problem. You've taken Diflucan before?"

"No," I said. "But I've used an antifungal cream a lot that had clotrimazole as the active ingredient, so I figure I tolerate the -azole family of antifungals fine. You know, fluconazole, Diflucan."

"Okay," he said. "That's fine. That makes sense."

I figured at this point that our business was done, but he wasn't reaching into his pocket for a prescription pad. Was there going to be a catch?

"So yeast," he said, settling back and getting comfortable in his armchair. "What else is going on with you?"

Was this some kind of joke? I looked him over for some sign that he was messing with me, but his face and body language looked open and sincere.

Why not? I thought. The guy asked what was going on with me. I should give him an honest answer.

"I have mercury poisoning," I said. "I got it from my amalgam fillings. I've been chelating using 25mg of DMSA taken at 4 hour intervals around the clock for three-day rounds. It's a protocol described by Andrew Hall Cutler in his book *Amalgam Illness*."

"Cutler, yes," he said. "I've heard of him. But who's prescribing your DMSA?"

"Nobody," I said. "You can just buy it on the internet."

"You can?" he laughed. "Wow. And you're just doing this on your own?"

"Yup."

"Are you taking any supplements?" he asked.

"Oh yeah," I said. "Lots."

"Like what?" he said.

The notebook with my supplement list happened to be in my bag, so I took it out, opened it to the page and handed it to him. In for a penny, in for a pound.

He looked it over.

"Why cayenne pepper?" he asked.

"I dunno," I said. "It was part of a bowel cleanse I did."

"Magnesium, yes. Flax oil, yes." He looked up. "Why no vitamin C?"

I explained about the bleeding hemorrhoid, and how blood-thinning C made it worse.

"It's so necessary, though," he said. "With heavy metal issues. Have you tried taking it in a different form? Something like Rose Hips. That would probably help your hemorrhoid, not make it worse."

"You're right," I said. "I hadn't thought of that."

"And your adrenals," he said. "Are you taking anything to support your adrenals?"

The conversation went on, we covered my adrenals, and then moved on to the theory behind chelation protocols. I started to really enjoy myself. I had never spoken to a real live human being before who understood what heavy metal toxicity was all about. He had even chelated some of his patients.

"I see it in my own patients," he said. "People do better on lower doses of chelators. It's got to come out slowly. So can I interest you in a DMSA challenge test?"

"No," I said. Cutler was adamant on this. Taking a large dose of a chelator just to see how much mercury came out in your pee was an easy way to get very very sick from redistribution.

"You can learn a lot from it."

"No thanks," I said.

"Okay," he said. "I respect that. I'm not going to push it on you. But how about some blood work? Just to see where everything's at."

I surprised myself by saying, "Yeah, okay."

He took a little pad out of his pocket.

"And here's your prescription for Diflucan," he said. "Five days. You're going to get some die-off, it can get quite intense, but if you can, see if you can make it through the whole five days."

He stood up, and before handing me off to the nurse for blood work, he paused and looked at me.

"Heavy metals are hard," he said. "But you're managing this really well. You're basically strong and healthy. I can see it, you're going to be fine."

I went to the nurse for blood work, and then stopped at the front desk to pick up a bottle of herbal adrenal formula and to pay my bill. I handed over hundreds of dollars that my health insurance would probably never cover. Still, it was worth it. I walked out to my car, fingering the prescription for Diflucan in my pocket, and thinking, I'm managing this really well, I'm basically strong and healthy, I'm going to be fine.

IV

❧❧

Flashes of Fantastic

As spring turned to summer, after 22 rounds of DMSA, my dump phase wound down, right on schedule. I felt some relief, my mercury symptoms were definitely less pronounced. It was good, I certainly wasn't complaining, but all that time I'd spent gazing at the graph of the dump phase, I'd hoped that my improvement would be more dramatic by the time I got to the bottom of the curve.

Physically, I could see improvements. I was now able to hold it together most of the time if I ate very carefully, took my supplements religiously, chelated like clockwork every other weekend, and avoided doing anything too taxing. My brain situation was improving too. My mood wasn't quite so steeped in darkness, and I was very occasionally able to attempt a little writing. I wasn't turning out anything good, of course. The part of my brain that was in charge of creativity had gone awol many months ago. And in general, I wasn't as smart as I used to be. I was slower, duller, much less fun to be around. But at least I was alive, I didn't feel like I was going to be destroyed at any moment.

The five-day course of Diflucan had been intense, but it had done its job. Around day four, I'd turned very pale with a hint of yellow and my liver had ached, but by the end of it, the yeast had been cleared from everywhere. My skin was completely free of the tinea versicolor fungal rash for the first time in ages. But the adrenal formula I got from the doctor didn't turn out so great.

It was obvious that my adrenals were in distress. I had several classic symptoms: excessive exhaustion after exercise, intolerance of foods high in potassium, salt cravings, inconsistent energy levels, and the 'adrenal silhouette': my curves had melted away and I was all bones and corners. I'd hoped that this adrenal formula would be different, but it was like every other adrenal remedy I'd ever tried. It boosted my energy some, but no matter how early in the day I took it, I ended up suffering from insomnia, too wired to relax and fall asleep. I gave up on it after a few days.

But I was happy with the rest of the help that the doctor was giving me. When I went back for my second appointment to hear the results of my blood work, I learned that I had low magnesium, low vitamin D, low B12, and low iron.

"I can mix you up a cocktail," he said. "Give them all to you at once, intravenously. It can take so long to get your levels up if you take them orally."

"Um, no way," I said. "What if I had a bad reaction to one of them? How would I know which one it was? At a really high dose? It sounds like a bad idea."

of a missed dose. I had done some retail research on-line and now was the proud owner of a stylish-looking chunky pink watch that you could program with eight separate vibrating alarms. I also had found a slim little travel clock that had an alarm that was ridiculously easy to reset. You could do it in your sleep, which was exactly what I needed to do.

I had my chelation routine down pat. I started at the same time every other week. Friday mornings, I took an empty clear pill minder and filled the first four compartments with my daytime chelation doses. M was the noon dose, T was the 3pm dose, W was the 6pm dose, Th was the 9pm dose. I donned my vibrating watch, and activated the alarms. Then I set the travel alarm for five minutes past noon. This alarm was the backup. If I failed to heed my vibrating alarm, this one would give me a second reminder to take my dose. This was especially important at night, when I sometimes slept through the vibrating alarm. And the clear pill holder was crucial to keep things straight at night too. In my sleepy dopey ALA state, I often woke up and asked myself questions like, *It's 3:02am, did I just take my dose? The backup alarm hasn't gone off yet, did I take the dose or not?*

A flick of the flashlight and a quick glance at the 3am compartment of the pill minder was all that was needed. If the capsules were in there, I hadn't taken them yet, if they weren't, I could go back to sleep, confident that I hadn't missed a dose, or accidentally taken it twice.

The mechanics of the rounds of chelation were pretty simple, but being on round with ALA was quite hard. I'd hoped that the dopey feeling would fade as the rounds went by. I'd had side effects on DMSA at first that had faded by the time three or four rounds had gone by. But ALA's effect on me was a stubborn presence that wouldn't go away. It faded a little bit, especially towards the end of rounds. Sunday evenings were often okay, but I never really felt good or comfortable when ALA was in my system.

I was pretty sure that the effect ALA had on my brain wasn't about the movement of mercury in my body. It was more to do with the chemical nature of ALA itself. Often, mercury toxic people had problems regulating a certain class of biochemicals in their system called 'thiols.' ALA was known to raise the body's thiol levels, as did many other ordinary substances like garlic and broccoli and milk. I'd never noticed having this kind of reaction to broccoli or milk, but the garlic capsules the dentist had given me had wrecked my head. It looked like I was slightly on the high-thiol end of the spectrum, and the concentrated thiol-raising power of garlic or ALA capsules was enough to push me over the edge.

ALA was raising my thiols, but it was also definitely moving mercury around my system. Every round seemed to knock a little bit of the stuffing out of me. I was left increasingly worn out, and the gains I got from taking vitamin C and getting B12 shots were more than wiped out. I got up and did things when I had to, I made a special effort to be up and about on the weekends when my girlfriend was home, but whenever I could, I conserved energy by resting in bed.

It certainly was a blessing that the dump phase was over, I didn't have to fight so hard to repress the voice of the mercury monster whispering in my head. But as ALA gradually scooped me hollow, I found that I didn't really have much going on inside me at all. I didn't have the energy and spark to think things up. My trains of thought didn't really go anywhere. They ran in circles, or just quietly ran out of steam. I didn't even have the oomph to find fault with my girlfriend and pick fights. Our relationship was peaceful, but it was a sad kind of peace. I got the feeling that I had been turned into a ghost, haunting my own life.

The hours and hours I spent in bed were hard to fill. Time crawled by, especially since my entertainment options were limited. I'd stopped enjoying listening to music, so that was out. When I listened now, even my favorite songs sounded empty. I couldn't define what was different, they all seemed to sound the same, but I found them to be more of an annoyance than entertainment.

Reading also had its difficulties. There were times when I propped a book up in front of my eyes, scanned the words, went through all the correct motions, but it just didn't take. It would feel incredibly tedious and exhausting to attempt to follow where the writer was going with all this.

My difficulties reminded me of a discussion I'd read in a writing book once, where the author had marveled at what we writers demand of our readers. We ask them to stare for hours at strings of tiny black marks on a page we have composed. And with only these very little prompts, we direct them to daydream up the rooms and people and telling glances and heartrending moments that we writers see in our heads. My brain often wasn't up for this momentous task. As a devoted and voracious reader, this was a particular hardship.

And still I chelated, staying steady on my course. No one said this was going to be easy. And no one said it was going to be quick. It seemed that two years was a good estimate of how long ALA chelation would take. I combed the boards for some idea of how it would go. Would I be hollowed-out and worn down for a year and eleven months, then I'd spring back all at once to my true shape? Or would it be a gradual filling-out, where the progress every day was slow, but I made it there in the end, inch by inch?

The truth seemed to lie somewhere between these two. People on the boards talked about long periods with no gains, and then after a year, hitting a turning point at 50 or 60 rounds of ALA. From my perspective of having completed 6 rounds of ALA, at the snail's pace of a round every other weekend, 50 or 60 rounds may as well have been as far away as the moon.

So I adapted to my new life. This was what I did now, I chelated. And did my best to fill the rest of my time. I bought the complete 85-episode run of the TV show *thirtysomething* on DVD and watched them all one by one on my laptop in bed. I'd watched this show back in Ireland as a teenager, around the time that I got my amalgams out. I'd loved it, but of course the lives of couples in their thirties living in America were very foreign to me. Now that I was a thirtysomething living in New York State, it should have reflected my experience, but I was no longer engaged in that life. Their struggles to build a career felt like something from my distant past. When the character Michael decided to be a writer, I laughed ruefully at what he went through. I had done that once. I had struggled to learn to write, but that had happened to another me. It was all gone now, swept away by the mercury. There was no way to tell if it would ever return.

Soon it was fall again, and my 34th birthday rolled around. I found myself looking back and taking stock as I often did at this time of year. It had been two years since I'd had my amalgams out, a year since I'd figured out I was mercury toxic and begun chelating. I had completed 30 rounds of DMSA in total, and nine of these rounds had included ALA. I was on my tenth round of ALA on my birthday. It felt more intense than recent rounds. I was more tired, unable to walk for any distance without needing to sit down, but at the same time I felt more peaceful and hopeful. Maybe it was the birthday nostalgia talking, but I felt like I was turning a corner, like something was going to change.

I was sitting on the bus going to work 36 hours after my birthday round ended. I was all prepared to feel like crap. Redistribution was due to hit, and I was ready to take whatever it dished out. But the fact of the matter was that I was feeling strong and energetic. I was sitting up straight in my seat, relishing the thought of spending the day engaged in physical labor.

The bus driver had the radio on, and was clicking through the stations, looking for a good song. He landed on one that caught my attention. It was utterly arresting. I was riveted by the music, it made me want to laugh out loud in delight. What was this exquisite masterpiece?

The chords seemed to progress perfectly inside my mind, making my emotions resonate with happiness. What was this song? Was it new? Was it old? Why had I never heard it before?

Halfway through the song, the bus driver clicked over to another station. I stared at him with my mouth hanging open. Was he crazy? I looked around, but the other passengers weren't raising an outcry.

It was then that I realized that the song wasn't special. It was just another piece of Lite FM fluff. Any specialness that was going on was happening inside me.

In the following days, it became clear that the round had shifted something inside my brain. Music sounded great again. And weirdly, some notes sounded a lot greater than others. That song I heard that morning featured a lot of bass notes that seemed to resonate with me. I couldn't find anyone else talking about this on the forums, but in the following months, some frequencies—even if they were generated by the rumble of a truck engine—sounded extra beautiful to me. And best of all, my ability to enjoy music was back. Permanently.

The return of music felt like a birthday gift. It was just the start of it. Every two weeks, I got another gift when I completed a round of ALA. My vision improved. Things had looked fine before, but suddenly, they were more crisp, like I'd traded in regular vision for HDTV. Then my hearing improved. My problem-solving skills returned. Everyday situations that used to baffle me were now easy to figure out. My night vision improved, and I became a better driver.

The best gift of all was when I got up one morning after a round, and sat on the porch watching the sunrise. I was able to appreciate the beauty with my crystal-clear vision. But it was nothing compared to the awesome miracle I suddenly experienced. I heard a witty remark inside my head. What a jolt. Then there was another one. Whoa! Next I thought up a funny little song. Oh my God! This hadn't happened in so long, but I remembered it now—I was a funny person!

In the following months it waxed and waned with the rhythms of chelation, but for hours, sometimes days at a time, the inside of my head became a fun place to be.

⟡

I continued to chelate, but after a few months the delightful surprises petered out. I knew now for a fact that ALA chelation absolutely and definitely worked, but what did it mean that I had made such progress after taking it for so few rounds? Was I well now? Was it over? Was the mercury gone?

Honestly, it didn't feel gone. Yes, the gifts I had been given were wonderful. I felt like I was being visited by parts of myself that I'd given up as dead. It was a profoundly beautiful experience to have a day where I sounded like my old self inside my head. But that was the problem. It was just a day or so here and there. Then the mercury clouds would gather, or I'd get on round again, and it was back to bed to watch *thirtysomething*.

I didn't begrudge them, my flashes of fantastic. I didn't want them to go away. But in a way, they made life harder to manage. I was up, I was down. I was a yo-yo at the end of a string, like I'd been during the dump phase.

Some days I felt so well, so vibrant in my mind, that I wondered why I wasn't looking for a job, making something of myself. Others, it was all I could do to heat up a frozen dinner and eat it in bed.

Still, my flashes of energy had to go somewhere. I decided that writing would be a good job to take on in my condition. I wouldn't have to get up and suit up and drive to the office every day. I could take things at my own pace, writing when I could, and putting it on hold on days when things were difficult. Things had gone so well for me on ALA, I wanted to spread the word about Frequent Dose Chelation. I decided I would explore the possibility of writing about it, and even talked to Andy Cutler, the author of *Amalgam Illness* about my ideas.

My energy got channeled into my relationship too. I began to talk to my girlfriend again. The silence was broken and I began to chatter to her about whatever was on my mind.

One night we were lying in bed falling asleep, and I noticed for the umpteenth time that the guys at the train station across the street had left the barrier down long after the train had left the station. The bells just kept on ringing minute after minute.

"Doesn't it bother you?" I asked my girlfriend. "The endless ringing?"

She lifted her head from the pillow. "I don't hear anything."

"At the barrier," I said. "Across the—"

It suddenly dawned on me that the ringing I was hearing wasn't loud enough to be the barrier.

"Oh my God," I laughed. "It's not real. All this time I thought it was across the street, but it was just ringing in my ears. I guess it gets quiet at night, so that's when I notice it."

"Doesn't that have a name?" my girlfriend asked. "Tintinitus?"

"Just one 'tin,'" I corrected. "Tinnitus. I think Tintin is a dog."

"No, that's Rin Tin Tin," my girlfriend said.

The conversation paused, and I closed my eyes, listening to bells that weren't really there.

"It's a terrible affliction," my girlfriend said. "Rintintinitus."

"Yes it is," I agreed.

"Constantly hearing dogs barking," she continued. "When they're not really there."

The two of us collapsed into giggles. A frozen place in my heart thawed out. How long had it been since we had made each other laugh?

❧

My girlfriend and I were speaking more, but I didn't really have a lot of material. Lots of my stories revolved around things people had said on the mercury forums, or clever ways I'd learned to control mercury symptoms.

One day we were driving somewhere, and she said she was going to make a quick stop at the gas station to buy an ice-cream bar.

"You should take chromium," I said. "It would even out your blood sugar and you wouldn't get sugar cravings."

She turned to me, anger written across her face and I was very surprised. I'd recently offered her lots of tidbits of advice like this, and she'd seemed happy to hear them.

"I am a human being!" she said. "I am not a jar of chemicals where you add a bit of this and a bit of that and make a perfect machine. I like ice cream! Normal people eat ice cream sometimes! And I get to decide when to eat it!"

"Sorry," I said. "I didn't realize I was being rude."

I analyzed this exchange. My girlfriend was a very tolerant person, so for her to turn on my like this must mean that I was being totally obnoxious without realizing it. Just because I felt better than I had before didn't mean that my ability to communicate like a normal person was restored.

I'd had months of practice at curbing the mercury monster's tongue. But now I saw that it wasn't just about keeping my mouth shut when I felt abysmal. All that mercury moving around my brain must have screwed up my social skills. It was now possible for me to start fights even when I was in a good mood. I resolved to redouble my efforts to monitor the appropriateness of what

I planned to say. It would be horrible to mess up my relationship now, after everything we'd been through.

I didn't say it to my girlfriend, but I knew that what she'd said was wrong. Human beings were jars of chemicals that could be fixed. And if I kept pouring ALA into my jar at regular intervals, hopefully the stuttering engine of my brain would kick into life and start running smoothly sometime soon.

❧

It was amazing the puzzles that became easy to solve during my flashes of fantastic. Back when I'd first started chelating, I'd tried to order a hair test. This was the best diagnostic tool to use for heavy metals because it gave more of an idea what was trapped inside cells rather than floating free in the bloodstream. I'd been told I wasn't allowed to order a hair test because New York State law forbade sending certain medical samples in the mail, and hair was one of them.

Back then, I'd given up on ever having my hair tested, but now I saw an obvious workaround. I asked a friend who lived over the border in Connecticut to order the hair test for me, and a few weeks later, I was sitting at my desk, printing out the full color heavy metal analysis of my hair.

The results were presented as a bar chart, and I first sought out mercury. It was very low, barely registering as a little bump on the graph. This didn't mean that all my mercury was gone. Mercury readings on hair tests didn't really have any bearing on a person's body burden. You could be thoroughly poisoned, your brain stuffed with trapped mercury, with none of it turning up in your hair. The true measure of mercury poisoning was whether the hair test met the counting rules showing deranged mineral transport.

I opened up Cutler's book *Hair Test Interpretation* to find the instructions for the counting rules, but before I began, my eye was drawn to another bar on the graph. It was the toxic element lead. My lead reading wasn't super-high, but it was there, and it was many times higher than my mercury reading. A conversation from the past echoed through my mind. My holistic dentist telling me I had mercury, yes, but many many times more lead.

I hadn't thought about lead in ages, not since I'd run through my apartment in the city, swabbing all the surfaces to see where I could be absorbing it from. I flipped through *Hair Test Interpretation* and read all the little sections that talked about lead.

It was an eye-opener. I finally understood how my system could be full of lead even though there were no sources of lead contamination in my home or environment. When large amounts of lead entered the body, only a fraction of it circulated in the bloodstream. The majority of it was stored in the bones. If a person showed high lead as an adult, there was no way of knowing for sure when they actually absorbed that lead. They could have picked it up at any point in their lives. Only by using detective work could they make a guess by identifying a time in their lives when they began to display lead symptoms.

My scalp began to tingle. I got the feeling that I was about to put together something big. There was always something that didn't sit right for me in my mercury history. My mercury exposure began in my teens when I got my amalgams placed. And yet, when I looked back over my childhood, I saw numerous little clues that pointed to mercury. How could that be? At first, I assumed that my mother had a mouthful of amalgam and passed the mercury on to me in the womb, but when I quizzed my sister about it, she reminded me that my mother hadn't had any fillings. When enough of her teeth had gone bad, she'd just had them all pulled and got dentures. The mercury content of any vaccines I got didn't explain things either. When I'd gotten my US visa, I'd had to produce my immunization record, and it was very patchy. In most cases, I'd had the disease rather than the vaccine.

My childhood 'mercury symptoms' couldn't have been caused by mercury. But could they have been caused by lead? What were the symptoms of lead poisoning? I looked them over and got goose bumps. Amblyopia or 'lazy eye' was mentioned about four times. I'd been prescribed glasses at the age of two in an attempt to correct my lazy eye. One of my earliest memories was being scolded for losing a new pair of glasses the very day I got them.

My other pre-amalgam 'mercury symptoms' all fit the lead profile. The chronic constipation I'd had all my life. The 'delicate stomach' I'd had. I couldn't count the number of times I'd been taken to the doctor because of unexplained stomach pains and vomiting. And why had I had Mee's Lines, white spots on my fingernails that were a sign of heavy metal toxicity all throughout childhood? Not because of mercury, I saw now, but because of lead.

I thought about my younger sister who had a lazy eye too. I thought about the fact that at the age of 5 she'd developed epilepsy, a brain disorder of unknown origin. Could it have been lead? Had our whole family been poisoned? I though about my father's epilepsy, my mother's diabetes, the atmosphere of unhappiness and dysfunction I'd grown up in. Could it all have been caused by lead? The family farm I grew up on certainly wasn't organic. Had anyone ever tested our water supply? Could it have been contaminated?

I let these questions hang. How could I ever be sure of where the lead had come from? All I knew for certain was that I was lead poisoned, and chelating with DMSA was taking the lead out as well as the mercury.

I turned back to my hair test. What would it tell me about mercury? Did my streak of amazing rounds so soon in ALA chelation mean that it was gone, that I wasn't as sick as I'd thought?

I went through the counting rules, and immediately, I met the first rule. Four of my essential elements were in the red zone. This meant that I had deranged mineral transport, I definitely had mercury toxicity, and would still have to chelate extensively with ALA to have any chance of making a full recovery.

It was validating to have a piece of paper in my hand that confirmed my diagnosis of mercury toxicity. But it was also sobering news. This thing was real, and I wasn't out the woods yet, not by a long shot. Mercury toxicity was a 'fringe' diagnosis, and hard to explain. I'd often heard myself or my girlfriend glossing over what was wrong with me, saying I 'just wasn't feeling well' or had 'food allergies' instead of launching into a long explanation why I couldn't come to an event or wasn't eating something. This habit had undermined the reality of my mercury diagnosis. I always believed it inside myself, I knew that my girlfriend always believed it, and people on the internet did too, but somehow it wasn't real outside of our home.

This hair test was independent confirmation that everything I was going through was real. It made me take myself more seriously. Instead of suffering through my mercury symptoms, I became more proactive in finding ways to support my health.

❧◈☙

My hair test yielded a wealth of diagnostic facts, the biggest one being that my thyroid was doing okay, but my adrenals were struggling. This was not surprising news, but hearing it from my hair test galvanized me into action. I was sick, I was going to be chelating for the foreseeable future. My body needed support to get me through this.

I went on the Frequent Dose Chelation Group and started reading posts about the adrenals. I'd always skipped these posts before because in my mind, there were only two treatment options for adrenal fatigue. On the one hand there were herbal formulae like the one my doctor had given me. I had tried these in so many forms over the years, and all of them made me wired and gave me insomnia. On the other hand, there was direct hormonal replacement of cortisol using prednisone or hydrocortisone. This was necessary for people whose adrenals were unable to perform. Cortisol was the hormone that gave people energy and the ability to withstand stress. I knew I was low. I knew I would benefit if I supplemented with it. But I hated the idea of the inevitable side effects. If I took supplementary adrenal hormone, my body's natural production of it would shut down. I would effectively be shutting off my adrenals for the duration of supplementation, with no guarantee that ending it would jumpstart them again.

I didn't want to do it, but I knew that all the other adrenal remedies didn't work. Was there no other option?

Reading through the adrenal posts online, I saw that there was something I had missed. There was a product called Adrenal Cortex, which was purely an adrenal glandular extract. It didn't provide any supplementary adrenal hormones, it didn't mess around with cortisol production, it just provided the building blocks for damaged adrenals to heal themselves. Dosing didn't need to be precise, side effects were rare, and a good guideline for tracking adrenal health was to keep a daily temperature chart. When body temperatures stabilized, and didn't fluctuate day by day, it showed that the adrenals were back on track.

I enjoyed taking my daily temperatures and seeing what they did. Just as the hair test had said, my thyroid was fine. My average temperature hovered around 98.6. If it had been lower, it would have indicated thyroid distress. But even though my average temperature was healthy, the daily and hourly fluctuations were alarming. In the morning I'd be 97.2, but late that afternoon, I'd have shot up to 98.8. There was no pattern to it, a line running through my graph was full of sharp peaks and valleys. But after a slow introduction of Adrenal Cortex, which caused no side effects except a mild case of mysterious itchiness for the first week, my temperatures started to converge. My graph got a lot smoother. I was also happy to note that it also showed the bump in temperature in the middle of my menstrual cycle that showed ovulation had occurred. In spite of all of the stress my body was going through, my ovaries were still functioning.

It wasn't just the temperature graph that showed improvement. My body let me know that Adrenal Cortex was really working. Used to spending a lot of my spare time in bed, it was a surprise to find that I no longer wanted to linger in bed in the mornings. I wanted to be up and about, getting on with the business of the day. The 3pm dip in my energy, which would often send me to my bed for a nap was now a thing of the past. And best of all, Adrenal Cortex didn't make me feel wired. When I lay down in bed at night to sleep, I slept, more soundly and deeply than I had in a while.

Adrenal Cortex was great, one of the most important discoveries I'd made on my chelation journey, but it didn't magically fix everything. I was still suffering through the dopey side effects on ALA, still feeling like a yo-yo at the end of a string as the rounds came and went. I almost could feel the mercury getting mobilized during rounds, and then getting shunted to another part of my body with redistribution. It was like a big game of musical chairs. One round would leave me feeling like my thyroid was suddenly burdened, then the next, it would be clear, but my thoughts patterns would feel more obsessive.

I hated that I could only chelate every other week, and that my rounds were bare-minimum short, but even after a second round of Diflucan, the yeast was just barely under control. I couldn't risk chelating more with DMSA, and I didn't want to play around with skipping it and trying ALA without it.

I was frustrated with how slowly things were going, especially when I looked out into the future and made projections of how long my recovery would take. I needed to complete 50 or 60 rounds of ALA. It was where people on the boards reported having their big turning points. For the average person, that represented a year of chelation. It really was the minimum that anybody could consider a complete course.

But at the rate I was going, chelating every other weekend, I was just completing 26 rounds a year instead of 52. To get to a grand total of 60 rounds of ALA and declare myself done, I would have to chelate for two more years.

This was hard to stomach. It was almost Christmas now, I had already chelated for a year, completing 35 rounds in total, but only 14 had included ALA. My chelation journey had gotten off to a late start, delayed for a year after my amalgams got removed because I hadn't even known I was mercury toxic. All in all, I was asking myself to live through a total of four years of sickness and instability, with unpredictable hours and days of horror and distress. Four years of not having a stable sense of self.

I was on round the next time I went into the city to see my therapist. I was lost in the ALA cloud, and telling her how hard it was on my relationship with my girlfriend.

"I don't know when I open my mouth," I said. "Who's going to come out. Dr. Jekyll or Mercury Hyde."

"Maybe you could be more gentle in the way you speak about yourself," she said. "You're sick, you don't feel good. Does that make you a monster?"

"No," I said. "You're right. It's not that interesting or dramatic. It's boring. It's just another tedious case of mental…" I groped through the ALA fog for a word that conveyed the meaning 'illness' but wasn't that word. Finally I gave up and just said it. "…illness."

My therapist just sat there and looked at me.

"What?" I said. "So I said it. Mental illness. I have a mental illness. So what?"

"You sound angry right now," she said. "Do you feel angry?"

I didn't say anything. I just glared at her.

"What are you feeling?" she prompted.

I looked at my watch, there was still 15 minutes left in the session.

"I feel like leaving," I said, gathering up my things.

I stood up to go.

"Perhaps we could—"

"Perhaps nothing," I said. "Not right now, not on round, not today. Some other time, maybe. But I'm not going to deal with this right now."

∼≈∽

And yet I was destined to deal with it. During one of my flashes of fantastic, my brain popped out a plan that would cut my projected two years of chelation in half. If DMSA wasn't in the picture, if there was something else I could take with the ALA to ease my mercury symptoms, something that didn't kill my immune system and exacerbate yeast, I could chelate faster. If I chelated for five full days every other weekend instead of just three days and two nights, I could move through chelation in double-quick time. I could be done with it all by next Christmas.

This magic other chelator that acted like DMSA but didn't cause yeast was not a figment of my desperate imagination. It existed, it was called DMPS, but I'd never even considered the possibility of taking it before because it required a prescription. Very few doctors knew enough about DMPS to feel comfortable prescribing it.

At first, I planned on getting it from my holistic doctor. I knew he'd prescribed DMSA, but had he ever mentioned DMPS? Maybe not. Maybe I'd go in there and spend a couple hundred dollars on a wild goose chase.

But then an even better idea came to me. In Seattle, there was a Nurse Practioner called Julie Anderson who specialized in helping people chelate using the Frequent Dose Chelation protocol. She wrote prescriptions for DMPS all the time. People from all over the country traveled to Seattle to see her. She had a very workable system of meeting with a patient in person once, and then having phone sessions with them from then on. She ordered blood tests for people through their local labs, and filled prescriptions through the mail. It would have been expensive to fly to Seattle just to see her, but I'd been planning to take a trip to Seattle in January anyway. It would all work out perfectly.

Being on the holistic end of things, she had reams of intake questionnaires that I needed to fill out and fax to her before our first appointment. One of the questionnaires was from a book by a brain expert called Daniel Amen. The quiz was used to determine which, if any, parts of a person's brain were malfunctioning and needed medication and support.

I asked my girlfriend to take the quiz with me. She would give me an outsider's perspective on my symptoms, and I was also curious to see how she scored herself.

On the first 14 questions of the quiz, I scored pretty low, a lot of 0s and 1s for Never and Rarely. They covered things like short attention span, disorganization, being unable to estimate how long things might take. They were all pretty much the opposite of what I was like.

But my girlfriend beside me was racking up the points.

"Procrastination?" I read. "My God, it's your middle name! Can you give yourself a 5? It only goes up to 4? Well, definitely give yourself a 4."

And then the quiz moved on to other brain areas, and the tables were turned.

"Has a tendency to hold onto own opinion and not listen to others."

"Ha!" my girlfriend said. "Give yourself a 4. You do that all the time."

"I do not!" I said. "I totally listen to others."

"You're doing it right now," she insisted. "Give yourself a 4."

"I am not!" I said. "You're just wrong. I'm going to give myself a 0."

After 40 or so questions, my girlfriend began to get restless.

"How long is this thing, anyway?" she complained.

She made it through another few questions, then shot to her feet, saying, "This is boring," and left the room. I looked at her scores. The only area she scored high on was ADD. It figured.

I finished the quiz and added up my scores. I was low on ADD, low on ADHD, but on each other area of the quiz, I scored very high. There was apparently something wrong with everything from my hypothalamus to my basal ganglia. This looked very bad. What did it mean?

I checked out the two Dan Amen books I found at the library and read them cover to cover. Here it was, right up in my face again, this idea that I had a mental illness. Scoring high in different areas of the quiz meant psychiatric diagnoses like OCD, borderline personality disorder, clinical depression. During all of my years of therapy, my therapist has refrained from diagnosing me. It was a policy that I had appreciated enormously. I didn't want a label, and I definitely didn't want to mask my true feelings by taking psychiatric drugs.

But now, besides my new symptoms that were clearly due to mercury like 'has low energy' or 'is frequently irritable,' there were things that I considered 'just me' chalked down as symptoms of mental illness. Some of them were problematic things that I had learned to work around like 'quick startle reaction' or 'tendency to freeze in anxiety-provoking situations.' But others were good. Weren't they good? What could be bad about being superorganized or punctual or enjoying routine?

But as I watched others around me, observing them from this new perspective, I could see the price I paid for my punctuality and neatness. Others didn't fret and obsess like I did. They could roll with change. They didn't need to know in advance everything that was going to happen that day, that week, that year. Trying to get some perspective on how severe my 'mental illness' might be, I asked my friend Gwen to fill out the quiz. She was someone I considered normal. Was the quiz designed so that even normal people would score high in some area, just because of their personality?

I watched Gwen fill out the quiz. "No," she kept saying. "Gosh, no, I don't have that." And I knew it was true, she wasn't lying.

I'd given positive answers to more than half the questions in the quiz. Gwen couldn't even scrape up 6 positive answers to the whole 71 questions.

So I was a bit mentally ill. So what? Mercury had ripped through me in the dump phase and rearranged some of my marbles. It was what mercury did after all, it was a neurotoxin.

But the realization slowly sank in that mercury wasn't just something that had screwed with my brain after amalgam removal. The self I'd had before I got my amalgams removed hadn't been normal, it had been poisoned by mercury too. Come to think of it, I'd probably never been normal. I'd been poisoned by lead from the start, my brain impaired from day one by toxic metals.

My trip to Seattle rolled around and I finally got to go to my appointment with Julie Anderson. I didn't hand over my Dan Amen brain quiz with the rest of my paperwork and she didn't ask for it. It was something I wanted to handle myself, I wasn't ready to talk about it. We talked through my history, and I was very curious to hear her thoughts on gluten intolerance. Was it curable? Was it something that might go away with chelation? She said that we could find out more if I took an IgG blood test. That kind of allergy was much more likely to clear up than celiac disease.

We talked about supplements I could try, EpiCor to boost my immune system, molybdenum which was highly recommended to help with mercury symptoms, and kelp to give a little boost to my thyroid. She phoned in my prescription for 25mg capsules of DMPS, and delivered a stern warning.

"If you start to get a rash, stop taking it right away!" she said. "In a small number of people it causes an allergic reaction called Stevens-Johnson syndrome. It starts with a rash, and ends up with your skin sloughing off."

"Ew, really?"

"Yes really," she said. "Keep an eye out for it."

I went home and when my DMPS arrived in the mail I tried out a weeklong round. I took it alone at first to see if I could tolerate it. My skin stayed intact, and I just felt extra tired after that first round. The next round was fine, I liked how DMPS caused much less redistribution than DMSA.

For my next round, I added in ALA, and started to stretch how long I took it for. I no longer had to limit my rounds to control the yeast. DMPS didn't have any effect on my immune system. I aimed for 5 days of ALA every other weekend, timed to overlap with my 7 day rounds of DMPS.

Things were mixed over the next couple of months. Julie ordered a set of hormone tests for me, and based on the results, I tried out DHEA and progesterone cream. It took time to sort out which of these new supplements were problematic and which were keepers. Molybdenum was awful, I couldn't tolerate it at any dose. Lithium seemed good at first, but I found that it made me tired as time went by. EpiCor was supposed to fix my immune system and banish the yeast, but instead, it made me have neuropathy and gluten-type reactions to beans and cheese, foods I'd never had a problem with before. DHEA made new hairs sprout on my chin, even at a tiny dose. At the end of it all, I just stuck with the Adrenal Cortex, occasional kelp for my thyroid, and progesterone cream to banish my menstrual cramps.

Reading Dan Amen's books had made me painfully aware of my nutty symptoms and what each one of them meant. The ones that seemed to damage my relationship most were the ones in the Cingulate Gyrus or 'overfocus' category. I was often uncontrollably anxious, single-mindedly obsessive, and over the past few months hadn't been able to change gears and vary my topic of conversation at all. I was a great big chelation bore.

If I was going to be honest, I had to admit that I couldn't handle change gracefully in any area of my life. I hated surprises, and stuck to my routine like glue. This made me good at chelating, a focused and productive writer, but didn't make me a lot of fun to live with, especially for my slightly ADD-esque girlfriend who liked to mix things up and enjoyed variety.

The worst part of my overfocus personality was that I used my girlfriend's 'flaws' to vent my anxiety. I turned my laser-like focus on whatever I perceived she was doing wrong, and wouldn't let up until she'd gotten a thorough understanding of how deeply she'd messed up. In the past, I'd thrown tantrums when she was ten minutes late for dinner, or had bought me the wrong kind of surprise gift. I hadn't been able to control the anxiety then, and I still wasn't able to control it now. I needed help.

The overfocus pattern was a mild form of Obsessive Compulsive Disorder. It was caused by low serotonin levels, and according to Dan Amen, would respond beautifully to SSRIs. I wasn't going to jump straight to taking Prozac, not after a lifelong personal stand against taking psychiatric drugs. But I did look very closely at Amen's supplement recommendations for people with low serotonin. The least side-effecty one seemed to be inositol, a relative of the B vitamins. I'd done badly on B3 so I worried about having a bad reaction. But then again I'd done wonderfully on B12, so maybe inositol would be great. I bought a jar of the powder, and the next day, took the recommended quarter teaspoon with my breakfast.

I didn't notice anything at first, maybe a slight sore throat. I went into my office and puttered around a bit, and then settled down at my computer to type up my daily to-do list. It was time to get to work.

I typed, *Go to the*

Then I found myself looking out the window at a bird in a branch.

store for potatoes, I continued.

Why had I paused? It wasn't like my brain was foggy or forgetful.

Do the

I picked up my paperweight and fiddled with it for a bit.

laundry.

Why was this going so slowly? My to-do list was something I banged out in sixty seconds unless I was feeling poorly and couldn't hold a thought in my head. But my head was totally clear. My next sentence was even sitting there, all ready to go. I started it.

Write 1,000 words on

But I just didn't seem to care very much about following through and getting the whole thing onto the screen. I kept on writing for a while, but this new mode of being my brain had entered was so strange and distracting. It was like my brain had turned into a wayward puppy, a distractible creature, uninterested in following my commands.

Wait. This was a familiar-sounding problem, but not because I'd ever experienced it. I jumped up to go find my girlfriend.

"I think I have ADD!" I told her. "I took too much inositol and now when I try to write, it seems just as important to look out the window!"

"Yeah that sounds right," she said.

"But I don't think I can control it!" I said.

"Looking out the window is fun," she said. "What's the problem?"

That dose faded, and over the next week or so, I found a more balanced effect on a much lower dose. It didn't change my personality, suddenly turning me into an easygoing person. But it took the edge off my obsessions, giving me a little more room to move and breathe.

It was around this time that the pain started. The morning after I ended my 40th round of chelation, I sat down in a chair and felt something give in my right hip. I tried to stand up, but the pain made me break out in a sweat. I sat for a while, waited, and then gingerly stood up. The throbbing pain faded after a while, but over the next weeks recurred if I did something as simple as bending down to tie my shoe.

And soon after that, a twitch began in my left eyelid. It felt like a flutter, and my vision would jump. At first I thought that others couldn't see it, but I was talking to my girlfriend one day and she said, "Whoa! What's up with your eye?" I tried to avoid eye contact with people when I could feel it happening.

The twitching was bad enough, but it soon grew into a dull ache under my cheekbone. This, on top of the hip problem was too much. I went for help.

Three days later, I was sitting in the local chiropractor's office making chit chat at the beginning of my first session.

"So what do you do?" he asked.

I told him I was a writer.

"Cool," he said. "What do you write about?"

"Mercury detox," I said. "Chelation therapy."

"Oh really?" he said. "Which kind?"

"Frequent Dose Chelation," I said. "It's based on a book by Andrew Hall Cutler called *Amalgam Illness*."

"Oh yeah," he said. "I've heard of that one."

"Really?"

"Yeah, there was this guy who used to come in, one of my patients, who kept telling me all about that stuff. Mega doses of Alpha Lipoic Acid and vitamin C, right?"

"Yup," I nodded and smiled. "How'd the guy do?"

"Oh, so-so," the chiropractor said. "He had a lot of problems. He swore by that protocol, though. He said it was great."

"It is," I agreed.

"And I'm sure it did make him feel better," he said. "I mean, it makes sense. Pour enough antioxidants down a person's throat and they're bound to feel better for a while. But after this dude stopped taking them, he went downhill again."

"Oh," I said.

I wondered what had gone wrong. Had he done it right? Had he gotten all of his amalgams out first? Had he made sure to chelate long enough? It was on the tip of my tongue to ask the chiropractor if he thought the guy had completed at least 50 or 60 rounds, but it was time to move on.

"Okay," the chiropractor said. "Why don't you hop up on the table and we'll see where we're at."

⊷⊷

My hip hurt more after my first session, but less after sessions two, three and four. I was able to hold the adjustments for longer and the pain was less frequent and not as sharp. Spring was in the air now, and the lease on our rental house was coming up for renewal. We were originally planning to buy a house in the area, but neither of us were in love with our sleepy rural village. My girlfriend and I sat down to discuss our options.

"Does living here make you happy?" my girlfriend asked.

I shrugged. Happiness wasn't something that I'd had much experience with since I'd left the city. Moving to this house had marked the beginning of my dump phase. I'd been sick for the whole two years we'd lived here.

"We need to do what makes us happy," she said. "What makes you happy?"

"Inositol?" I said.

"What else?"

I stared blankly at her.

"What are you dreams?" she asked. "What do you want to do in this life?"

That one was easy.

"To chelate," I said. "To get well."

"And?" she prompted. "Besides that?"

I shrugged. That was pretty much the focus of my whole life.

"I'm trying to find out if we should stay here," she explained. "Or if we'd be happier somewhere else."

"We could really move?" I said. "To a whole other place?"

"We can at least think about it," she said.

We got out the map of the Metro North train lines. We crossed off all the undesirable places: all of Westchester, large cities, the richest towns in America, anything sited on a toxic waste dump, and towns we just plain didn't like. There were four places left. One was called Beacon.

"Then we should move to Beacon," I said. "Someone said I'd like it there."

"Who?" my girlfriend said.

"Some woman," I said, grasping at an incomplete memory. "I can't remember who. She seemed very sure of it."

"Do you know anything about Beacon?" my girlfriend asked.

"Nope," I said. "But I can look it up."

Over the next few weeks, I thought about the life I was leading in this house. Most of my time was spent alone. The only people I came in contact with were my girlfriend who I saw when she wasn't at work, my therapist who I saw twice a month, and my girlfriend's father who dropped by for tea once in a while. Then there were friends like Gwen, the couple over the border in Connecticut, and one other couple who lived an hour away. These friends I saw maybe once every month or two. I had the people I saw on Tuesdays at the farm program, and that was pretty much literally all the people I had in my life. It was pathetic.

I did some research about Beacon. It was on the river, right on the train line to the city, but half an hour closer than we were now. There was a big art museum there, and from the looks of the town's social networking site, half of Brooklyn's artists had migrated up there to enjoy the arty vibe. There were listings of social events, film screenings, board game nights, life drawing classes. It all looked like such fun. And the perfect place to start up a writing group.

As soon as I had that thought, I couldn't let it go. I began to daydream about a whole other kind of life. One where I spent time with actual people, sitting around in coffee shops discussing our novels in progress. My girlfriend and I would host dinner parties. I'd go to board game nights. I'd spend my time at home during the day writing, but then at night, my social life would be full, there would always be someone to call, friends to hang out with.

My vision felt a bit delusional. When was the last time I'd made a friend? Really, on my own, without my girlfriend's help? Did I honestly think that I could commit to starting a writing group while still chelating? Who would want to hang out with me, with my diseased over-focused mind and tired chelating body?

I don't care, I thought. I want this. I want to have a normal life again. I'll do what it takes. I'll learn how.

I could see a road dividing in front of me with two options. All I'd done recently with my life was sit around and wait. I could either hide away in this house for the next few years, hoping that normality would be visited on me one day by the chelation gods, or I could make normality happen, I could go out and build the best life I could with the hand I was dealt.

I thought about the hand I had been dealt. My brain was still clearly impaired, but I wasn't tortured like I'd been during the dump phase. I wasn't mentally shut down like I'd been during the first year of chelation. I had lots of thoughts and feelings, they just were a bit crazy sometimes.

If I was going to live a real and normal life, I decided that I had to stop being afraid of myself. I had to stop shutting down what was going on inside me. I couldn't keep closing the door on every negative or 'crazy' thought or feeling I had. I had to accept them and work with them. Non-mercury-toxic people sometimes had 'crazy' feelings too, and they lived with them and expressed them.

Heck, most mercury toxic people expressed their crazy thoughts and feelings all the livelong day and nobody batted an eyelid. I'd BEEN one of those mercury toxic people once, back in the city before I'd gotten my amalgams removed.

Well the time for change had come. If we were moving to a new house in a whole new town, then it was time to stop treating my mind like a can of socially toxic fumes. It was time to be myself, even if that self was a bit sick, and deal with the craziness as it came up. It was time to get out there and meet people and make friends and learn how to live a normal life.

V

❧

Rebuilding

We went to check out Beacon and instantly fell in love with it. I looked for houses to rent and made an appointment to go see one, an elegant Victorian a short walk from the train station and Main Street where all the shops were. The landlord, an artist, gave us the tour, and one bright airy room upstairs caught my writer's heart.

"This would be my office," I said immediately.

"What?" my girlfriend said. She hadn't even made it into the room yet.

"This one's mine," I said. "You can't have it."

"Oh, fine," she said.

My only misgiving about the house was all the climbing I would have to do. Unlike our old house, this one had stairs. And was situated at the top of a very steep hill. And besides that, there were two sets of steep outdoor stairs to climb to get to Main Street. When we left the house and took a stroll over to Main Street to look at the health food store, I huffed and puffed, hauling myself up the stairs. And then there was long, long Main Street to get down. It was nice to have everything within walking distance, but that actually meant doing some walking.

I was glad that there were benches strategically situated all along Main Street, and I eagerly flopped down onto one to rest as we made our way to the store. Once there, I made a mental list of all of the gluten free goodies I would buy once we moved in. I didn't know how I would make it up that final hill to the house carrying a bag of shopping, but there was parking all along Main Street. It wouldn't be weird if I drove everywhere.

Packing up the whole house for our move was easy on good days and hard on bad days. I either whipped through 25 boxes in an afternoon, or struggled to get done with even one. But it all got done in the end, and the movers came and dropped it all off at the other end, and the long process began again, but in reverse. I was aware now of my girlfriend's ADD issues, and having more energy than I'd had in a while, I took charge of the unpacking process. I wanted us to unpack right this time. I wanted us to resist the urge to just plop things in the first place that came to mind. I wanted this new house to be organized, to be as close to perfect as possible.

I had counted all of the boxes, and had added up my estimates of how long each organizational task would take. If we worked efficiently, there were a few short weeks of work ahead of us. But of course my girlfriend's amazing powers of procrastination could turn that into months.

I laid it all out for her, explaining that we needed to focus.

"So I can't do anything except go to work and unpack?" she said.

"That's right."

"But I want to go to the library," she said.

"No, you can't."

"Where can I go?"

We brokered a deal where she was allowed to go to the grocery store, hardware store, and the bank, but only if necessary.

"Just make sure you unpack at least ten boxes a day, alright?" I said.

"That's a lot of boxes," my girlfriend grumbled.

"You'll benefit from this too," I said. "Don't you think it'll be good for you to have a house that's really organized?"

"Fine, fine," she said, walking away.

We barely had time to speak to each other over the next few weeks. We spent every free moment unpacking and working on the house. I kept an eye on my girlfriend, making sure that she was doing her share and doing it right. The house was shaping up nicely, but we still had a ways to go. I wondered how long until my girlfriend would tire of all this and start shirking her duties.

Things came to a head with the fish soup. I couldn't understand why my girlfriend had arrived home with two pounds of frozen hake one day. She was a vegetarian and hadn't eaten fish in sixteen years.

"It was leftover from my boss's Seder," she said. "I think I know what I want to make…"

165

She continued to go on about the fish and how she was going to cook it, but I could see that this was some kind of procrastination ploy on her part. We were supposed to be unpacking, not messing around with fish she probably didn't even want to eat. A couple of days passed, and I decided to take care of the fish myself, and turned it into a quick soup.

My girlfriend came home in the middle of the cooking.

"What are you doing?" she asked.

"Making fish soup," I said.

"But I told you I was going to cook that fish!" she said. "I have a recipe! We had a long conversation about it!"

"We did?" I said, guilt washing over me.

"Don't you remember?" she asked. "We went back and forth and then we finally decided we'd cook it together. I was really looking forward to it!"

I didn't remember. When I tried to recall conversations about the fish, all I got was my own voice-over, *Get rid of the fish so we can unpack, unpack, unpack!*

My girlfriend stormed out of the house and sat on the porch and didn't speak to me for the rest of the long evening.

The rest of the weekend went pretty much just as badly. When we were working on setting up the garden, my girlfriend said how she was planning to plant corn, beans and squash in the 'three sisters' formation by the back fence, but with perennial versions of the plants that she'd have to find online and get shipped to us. I was wise to this kind of ADD talk. Lots of my girlfriend's 'plans' never came to fruition.

"So is this something you're going to do for real?" I asked. "Or should I have a backup plan for that part of the garden?"

She exploded.

"I am sick of you," she spat out, "and your need to piss in every corner of this house! We have been unpacking for three solid weeks! I have had enough of your controlling and nitpicking! I'd rather be alone that deal with this kind of attitude!"

It was a horrible shock to experience such anger from someone who was usually so calm and accepting. I ran into the house and locked myself in the bathroom and had a good cry. Why had things gone so horribly wrong?

It was tempting to blame it all on mercury, to say that the mercury monster had caused this fight, and if I just zipped the lip and kept the monster under control, everything would be fine. But the truth was, there was no mercury monster. There was just me. I had to take responsibility for what I'd done.

I was rusty at this, I could almost hear the hinges in my brain creak as I approached my girlfriend later that night and said, "We have to talk."

It was scary to talk to her about my negative feelings. Was this going to destroy everything? Even though I cried a lot during the conversation, it didn't feel like a hopeless descent into mentally ill misery. It was a true communication of how I felt. I could feel her at the other end of the line, understanding me, hearing me. And when she spoke, I listened hard.

"You have to stop bossing me around," she said. "And I want no more of that mechanistic bullshit about what vitamins you want me to take. It's all you ever talk about. I accept other people for who they are. I never ask you to change. Can't I have even a fraction of that attitude returned to me?"

It dawned on me how poorly I'd listened to her, what a bad partner I'd been. Yet in the end, I felt closer to her than I had in a long time.

❧

As the rounds passed, my body felt stronger. After the unpacking push, I didn't need to take a week in bed to recover. I kept going. I happily trotted up and down all the stairs and hills that I'd worried about when we first moved in. One day, I even surprised myself by wanting to run up a flight of stairs. It was fun. There was a spring in my step that I hadn't felt in ages. My body was definitely getting well. It was just my mind that still needed some help.

One good conversation with my girlfriend didn't make everything better. I struggled in this new place of taking all of my feelings seriously, both good and bad.

Sometimes something upsetting would happen, and I would feel awful! And I was expected to sit with this feeling and process it and write in my journal about it and act on it? Sometimes it went on for hours, days. How could a person feel this bad about trivial nonsense for so long? It had to be the mercury talking. But I held on, and eventually it always passed, and I felt glad that I'd stuck it out.

All through that first summer in Beacon, I worked on making a healthy connection with my feelings. It was a summer when my girlfriend was away for a month traveling with her family, and then another month for work. This was good, because I got to practice being around some difficult feelings without having to interact with anyone. But being left at home so much didn't make me happy.

When she came home from her second trip, I told my girlfriend, "We have to talk."

I wanted to share my true feelings with her. The biggest of these feelings was anger. I cried and berated her for neglecting me, for not including me in her plans, for seeing me as some sick appendage she could just park at home while she went off having fun.

I couldn't let it go. I was so unhappy, and needed to make her unhappy too. After a long fight where it felt like nothing was resolved, just bad feelings dumped all over her, I began to despair. How could this help? I was poisoning our relationship. I should zip the lip and let it go.

"Bet you wish I'd go back to the way I was when I was sick," I said. "When I was quiet and just stayed out of your way and didn't badger and harangue you."

"No," she said. "I wouldn't want to go back to that for one second."

"Why not?" I said. "It wasn't like you were the one who was sick."

"I wasn't sick," she said. "But do you think it was fun for me? Right now, you're totally crackers, you're a great big pain in my ass, but at least you're not ignoring me. Do you know what it's like to live with someone who's sick and miserable and won't talk to you?"

I shook my head.

"It's not good," she said. "Not good at all."

Things were slowly getting better inside my home, but there was the wide world to contend with too. Living in Beacon, there was always something going on, several nights a week. I had more social engagements in one month than I'd had the whole two years I'd been sick. I started the writing group I'd dreamed about, and we met every week at a local wine bar. Besides that, there was the book club, the science fiction book club, gallery openings, two different board game nights, and best of all, dinners and parties at the houses of the circle of awesomely cool lesbians we had met since we'd arrived.

I found myself drawn to the kinds of people I would have considered 'above me' or 'too together' before. Back in the city, I had made a lot of friends who had been sick in one way or another. We'd had a lot in common, and looking back, I suppose that that thing was mercury poisoning. But now I didn't want to seek out people who were sick. I had nothing to learn from them. I wanted to befriend healthy people. I wanted to spend time with them, to let them model to me how people behaved whose lives weren't ruled by mercury. They seemed happy to welcome me into their lives, and I took notes on what 'normal' looked like these days.

One of the first things I did to fit in a little more was to stop taking the jumbo old-lady pill minder with me when I went out to dinner. I rearranged my regimen so that I took the bulk of my supplements with breakfast, and any twice-a-day extras with lunch, plus a top-up at bedtime. It was weird enough that I was always the only person at the table who was gluten free. I wanted to be able to sit in a restaurant with the book club and not have to also explain about my supplements.

It felt very freeing to appear more normal, but as more long rounds of ALA went by, my brain seemed to be taking a turn for the worse. I had met a lot of new people over the summer in Beacon, and I now feared being in situations where I would have to introduce people to each other. I was having a problem recalling people's names. I hadn't forgotten them, I just couldn't bring them to mind fast enough to be useful.

Parties began to be stressful to me. The writing group got harder too. People's names weren't the only problem, now ordinary words seemed harder and harder to summon. I felt like I was beginning to sound like a half-wit.

I sat at a party once beside my girlfriend, talking to another couple.

"I hate that thing," I said. "You know, that thing where you can't say the words?"

"What do you mean?" my girlfriend asked.

"There's a word for it," I struggled. "Where you can't choose the right words, and you're all stupid-sounding."

"Oh, you mean 'inarticulate,'" one of the women said, laughing.

"Thank you," I said. "I hate that I'm so inarticulate."

"Oh you're funny," the other woman said. "What's the word for when you can't find the word," she mimicked. "Too cute!"

I knew she thought I had been joking, and I laughed along, but the tedious truth was that it wasn't a joke.

The months went by and I began to wonder if this was just how chelation worked. As my body grew stronger and more resilient, I paid the price by having my mental faculties eaten away. I tried not to worry about it too much. Whatever this thing was, it wasn't making me depressed or unhappy, it had just turned me into a total airhead.

❧

I was making a lot of progress making friends with normal people. My girlfriend and I started getting regular invitations to eat at people's houses. We always accepted, but then came the awkward negotiation where I tried to gauge their interest in really learning about gluten. It was a hidden ingredient in so many foods. It was so easy to contaminate a dish with it while cooking. I really didn't like asking these people I barely knew to do all this work just for one little dinner.

And was there really a need for me to keep eating gluten free? What if it wasn't an issue for me anymore, but I just didn't know it?

The IgG allergy test Julie Anderson had ordered for me when I'd seen her in Seattle had come back negative for gluten. But this didn't mean that I was in the clear. There were all kinds of different ways that the immune system could be damaged, resulting in a gluten allergy. Celiac disease apparently generated a whole other set of antibodies, and these could be detected in a different blood test. I was curious to see if I'd come up positive if I took this one. I spoke to Julie about it on the phone.

"The celiac blood test is pretty accurate at testing specifically for the presence of celiac antibodies," she said. "I can order it for you."

"That would be great," I said.

"But you do realize," she said, "that you're going to have to eat gluten beforehand to produce the antibodies. Being strictly gluten free for a long time means they've cleared out of your system."

"Yes, I know," I said. "Do I have to eat it for more than one day?"

"No!" she said. "Just once. Just a little will cause enough of a reaction. Take it easy, okay?"

Two days before the blood test, it was very very strange to open up my girlfriend's box of Wheat Chex and actually touch it on purpose. I generally avoided touching other people's gluten in case invisible crumbs stuck to my fingers and made their way into my system.

I took one little square of cereal and put it in my mouth, resisting the urge to wipe my hand on my shirt to get the hidden gluten crumbs off. Nothing could stop the contamination now, the wheat was inside me. I chewed the little gluten bomb, blown away by how incredibly *wheaty* it tasted. It was a flavor I hadn't encountered in years. Mercury must have erased my 'wheat' file, it tasted so weird and foreign to me now.

I went on with the rest of my day, feeling fine, but knowing in the back of my mind that bad things were on their way. My usual pattern was to not feel any gluten symptoms until the morning after I ate it, so I didn't make any sudden moves when I woke up. I braced myself for a foul mood, neuropathy, tunnel vision, everything I'd experienced the last time I'd been glutened. How bad was it going to be? Was it going to be worse, as the literature on celiac disease suggested it would be, symptoms increasing in severity the longer a person refrained from eating gluten? Or would my secret hope be realized? Would chelation have done its magic and freed me of this terrible burden of gluten intolerance?

I sat up. I turned my head, wiggled my fingers and toes.

And laughed.

I felt fine. My mood was fine. My vision was normal. I stood up and walked around. Yes, if I paid attention, I noticed a little neuropathy in the fingers of my left hand. Nothing too alarming, just a slight numbness. And the left side of my scalp felt a bit funny too. It wasn't quite a headache, it wasn't quite numb, it was just an odd sensation that made me aware it felt different to the rest of my head. And that was it.

I felt the tiniest hint of disappointment that I wasn't a hundred percent cured, but mostly, I felt very very grateful. This was such an enormous improvement.

I wasn't going to rush out and start eating gluten again, but if this was all it was going to do to me, I didn't have to live in terror of it anymore. I could relax about eating at people's houses. Even if someone screwed up and contaminated my food, it wouldn't be a big deal.

The result of the celiac blood test came back. It was negative.

"That doesn't mean you can eat gluten," Julie Anderson warned.

"I know," I said.

"As long as you're having symptoms, you should stick

with the gluten free diet."

"I know."

I still had no idea how gluten was affecting my immune system. And yet I felt very cheerful about my progress. Chelation had made 95% of my gluten symptoms go away. Maybe one day, when chelation was done, I'd make it all the way to a 100%.

The gluten mystery remained unsolved, but the case of the inarticulate foggy-brained lesbian got cleared up the following month. I was reading about copper toxicity, something that often went along with heavy metal poisoning. Because of liver problems, mercury toxic people often ended up retaining too much copper. The symptoms of copper toxicity and mercury toxicity were practically indistinguishable, except for the fact that in women, copper toxicity caused PMS. Taking vitamin C, and especially zinc with meals was a sure-fire PMS remedy. The zinc competed with copper in the gut for absorption, automatically lowering its levels.

I found this information interesting. It was something that every woman should know. It wasn't relevant for me, because my PMS days had ended the moment I'd had my amalgams removed. Suffering through two days of foggy-brained misery every single month was a thing of the past.

Or was it?

I scrabbled through my papers and took out my latest temperature chart. I counted up the days since my cycle had started, took out my diary and correlated the dates. This month, yes, I'd had an emotional drama that had seemed very important at the time, but had resolved itself with the arrival of my period. And last month too, I'd had those couple of tearful days that fell right before my period started. And all of this spaciness that had been going on for months. Could it be? Was it possible that it wasn't mercury, but copper?

Of course it was. I'd been chelating hard with ALA for months. People who chelated intensely with ALA had to keep an eye on their copper levels, because one of the side effects of ALA was a tendency to hold onto copper. How had I forgotten that? And a few months ago, I'd gone and stopped taking my supplements with dinner, absorbing extra copper because the supplements didn't compete with it for absorption. No wonder my copper levels had gone so high.

Fixing copper toxicity was very easy. Taking vitamin C and zinc with meals would clear it up in a month or so. But I was tired of being pulled through the wringer. I'd just passed the threshold of 100 days of ALA chelation. I decided to take a couple of rounds off to let my copper levels fall.

Going off ALA was daunting. I was at round 54 now. I had chelated like clockwork every other weekend since the 'autistic' fiasco in London at round 18. I decided it would be safer not to stop chelating entirely. I would continue as usual taking DMPS without the ALA.

I kind of held my breath through that first round when I was skipping ALA. But I didn't experience any ill-effects. In fact, I started to feel great. The excess copper started to clear out of my system, and suddenly, I felt fine. I could think clearly, remember effortlessly. I wasn't a woolly-headed inarticulate mess anymore. I took a second round off, and the clarity continued. I reveled in my smartness, and couldn't help crowing over the ass-kicking I dealt out when we played Scrabble at board game night.

When it was time to go back on ALA, it chafed terribly to return to the inevitable spaciness. But intellectually, I knew that I was doing the right thing. I would thank myself later for making this sacrifice. I just had a few more months to go before crossing the threshold of 150 days of ALA chelation. It would only be 40 rounds of ALA chelation for me, but because most of my rounds that year had been supersize 5-day rounds, I had started counting days instead of rounds. 150 days was my shining goal, my equivalent of 50 regular-sized rounds, the threshold I had been pining to cross since I'd started ALA chelation 18 months before.

❧ ❧

I was still taking my trips into the city every other week to see my therapist, but even though the train journey was shorter, I began to resent the time it was taking away from my writing and the rest of my busy new life. I'd begun to wonder why exactly I was going all the way into the city and paying all this money to see her. Now that my head had cleared, it seemed like the only thing that was wrong with my life was that I was chelating. Everything else was the best it had ever been. Did I really need to pay someone a hundred and fifty dollars to hear how my life was going well? I liked my therapist a lot, but I figured that one of these days, I was going to have to give her the boot.

The next time I went into see her, I was on round, feeling the all-too-familiar feeling that I was trapped in a well, physically walking among the normal people, but miles away from them in my own mercury world.

"I know it's not true," I said, "But it feels like I've felt like this forever."

She nodded.

"It's like a day, an hour in this place takes forever," I said. "No. It's more like this place exists in another time, not the time that ordinary people occupy. And I have days in that ordinary time too. But then I come back here again, and it's eternal."

"I think what you're describing is a thing called state memory," she said. "When you move into a certain state, you can't access the memory of 'ordinary time' as you call it. So every time you're in there, all you can remember is what it felt like to be there the last time you were there, and the time before, and before that. So it feels eternal, even if it objectively lasts for a very short time."

"Yes," I said. "Exactly. That's what it is. State memory."

"So, you seem to be doing well in your new home, doing your writing…"

I nodded.

"…and making new friends."

I nodded and smiled.

"It feels like a new phase is beginning for you," she said. "Something more stable. And I wondered what direction you wanted to take things in here. In your sessions."

Oh boy, here it was, the moment I'd been putting off.

"We could work on the memory states you're finding yourself in," she said. "Like right now."

I sighed, and tears began to flow out of my eyes.

"What came up there?" she asked.

I opened my mouth, but it took a moment to frame the words.

"I'm not going to work on those states," I said. "Here with you. Chelation ends soon, the states will end along with it."

"It may not be that simple…" she began.

"Listen to me," I said, crying harder. "What I'm trying to tell you is that this is it. For now. This is our last session."

180

Tears sprang up in her eyes too. Our bond was deep. She may not have understood every nuance of what my sickness meant, but she'd been a witness to it. She had sat with me through the worst.

"I'm not sick anymore," I said.

It was terrifying to make such a bold statement. But I truly meant it. Physically, mentally, emotionally, chelation had changed everything. I was no longer an injured bird that needed her care.

"I know I'm not perfect," I said. "But I can do this. I know I can live my life. Like a normal person. You know?"

"I know," she said, and wiped her eyes. "And you know my door is always open. Just call and you can come back any time. I would love to see you."

"I know," I said.

She stood up. "Let me give you a hug?"

I fell into her arms and wept some more. And then I dried my eyes, blew my nose, and went out and began my new life as a normal person.

Two days later, it was my birthday. I was thirty five years old. It was a year since I'd had that miraculous round where music had returned to my life, when I'd known for sure that ALA worked. Two years since the darkest days of the dump phase, when I'd reached out and found the stories of other mercury toxic people and begun to chelate.

I spent my birthday with my girlfriend at a baseball game. We were neither of us big fans, but she'd gotten free tickets at work, and it sounded like a fun day out. Except of course, I wasn't having any fun. I was on round, and ALA's effect on my brain seemed especially strong. I sat in my seat, far above the field, and pretended to be engrossed in the game so that I wouldn't have to navigate the conversation going on between my girlfriend and her co-workers.

But in reality, I wasn't following the game at all. I was struggling because ALA was distorting my perception of reality. When I looked at the field, I couldn't shake the belief that I was watching the game on a screen. Reality had become kind of flat and two-dimensional. This had happened to me before, but it hadn't been this strong. The effect was magnified when I looked up at the actual screen that the game was being shown on. I tried to break the spell by putting my head down and closing my eyes.

"Are you okay?" my girlfriend asked.

"I should take a walk," I said. "Come with me?"

We navigated the steep steps, and spent some time walking back and forth between the snack food vendors and the bathrooms.

"I'm sorry," I said. "Would it be okay if we went home?"

"Don't apologize," she said. "It's your birthday, not mine."

"I just hate this," I burst out. "It's horrible!"

"Poor pet," she said. "But it will pass soon, right? You'll be fine again in no time."

She was right. The next day, I felt much more grounded, and by the time the round ended, I was totally fine. But it bothered me that just a couple of months from my arbitrary finish line, I was still having intense chelation symptoms.

That wasn't how it was supposed to go. On the Frequent Dose Chelation protocol, there was no official number of rounds that a person was supposed to complete. The guideline was that chelation should continue six months past the point that ALA provoked no more mercury symptoms on round. I suspected that most of my reaction to ALA had more to do with its high thiol content than any mercury it was stirring up, but chelation should normalize my thiol levels too, ending those symptoms. I was nowhere near symptom-free, and yet I was planning soon to stop. Was I being stupid? Maybe the arbitrary finish line of 150 days on ALA was a bad idea.

Near the end of my next round, on my 110th day of chelation with ALA, I woke up feeling a little itchy.

Maybe this is it! I thought. Maybe this is finally the Stevens-Johnson syndrome that Julie Anderson talked about!

The thought filled me with glee. I examined my skin to see if it was showing any signs of sloughing off, but to my disappointment it was totally intact and blemish free.

Nevertheless, I launched into an elaborate fantasy where I called up Julie Anderson in distress.

Oh Julie, I'd say, *I really really really want to keep on chelating, but I think I'm starting to have a reaction to DMPS.*

Then you must stop! Julie would say. *Stop chelating now! Forevermore you must stay away from DMPS and all other chelators! Do you understand me? Never chelate again!*

But my itchiness faded away, and I got up and started my day of work.

As I wrote, my mind began to wander and I started thinking about my girlfriend. The fact that I was chelating had an effect on her life too. It wasn't just about me. Was it fair to subject her to all of these alarms in the middle of the night? Make her leave the baseball game early? Ask her to do all the driving when I felt spaced out?

Maybe I should call her up at work and tell her that I was willing to stop chelating right now for the sake of our relationship.

I caught myself and gave myself a little mental shake. This was ridiculous, I had to snap out of it. But the truth was that I couldn't. It kept surfacing in my mind in different forms, this nagging thought that I needed to quit chelating.

Okay, I thought. I'm not going to suppress this train of thought, I'm going to engage with it and process.

Hello little train of thought, I said to myself. *Why should I quit chelating now? Why today?*

Why two months from now, in December? it countered. *It's all arbitrary. Quitting in October versus quitting in December, who cares? Nobody is watching.*

I turned this idea over in my mind for the rest of the day. Was this train of thought voicing something negative? Was it speaking from a place of sickness, should I ignore it? But what if it was perfectly reasonable? What if it was making perfect sense?

It seemed like a revolutionary idea, to change a deadline that had been set in stone for so long. Was I ready to abandon the idea of the 50 or 60 round golden turning point? How could I expect the recoveries that other people had seen if I didn't chelate as fully as they did? I had busted a gut over the past year to squeeze in as many days as I could on ALA. But my 110 days still only represented forty something standard-sized rounds. What if I stopped and it turned out that I wasn't really done? What if it was a terrible mistake?

I thought about my therapist, not because I wanted to call her up to ask her what to do. Instead, I turned over the memory of the last thing she said to me. *You can always come back. My door is always open.* I knew that she was going to say those words even before they came out of her mouth. It was one of the things that made it possible for me to stop seeing her. Quitting therapy was never a forever decision. If I needed her, she was there.

I realized that chelation was the same. If I quit now, it didn't have to mean that I would never chelate again. If the mercury symptoms returned, chelation was always there for me. I could pause chelation for six months and see what happened. If it was clear at that point that I needed more, then I'd go back on round.

It was then that I picked up the phone and called my girlfriend. I ran the plan past her to see if it sounded reasonable. Did she think I was just being a quitter?

"How long have you chelated for?" she asked me.

I cast my mind back. I'd begun chelation soon after I'd turned 33. "Almost two years," I said. "I guess it will be two years in a couple of weeks."

"And how many rounds have you done?" she asked.

This information was sitting right in front of me in my planner.

"This is round 60," I said. "But I haven't done 60 rounds of ALA. That's really the only kind of chelation that counts."

"It doesn't matter," she insisted. "You have chelated like a dog for two years. You absolutely deserve a break. Your plan is a good one. Okay?"

"Okay," I smiled.

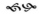

And so I stopped. The first weekend off chelation coincided with a visit from family. My sister, her husband and two children came from London to spend Halloween with us. My girlfriend and I had the week planned out: the local Halloween Parade, pumpkin carving, apple picking for the kids. A screening of the Rocky Horror Picture Show, and nights out at some nice restaurants with good gluten-free menus for the adults.

We went all-out, ran around having a good time. It was a great visit. On the last night, my sister sat in the living room with me and my girlfriend, quizzing us about our travel plans. She was always going somewhere herself, and liked to rope other people in too whenever she could.

"Well," my girlfriend said, "We were sorta talking about going to New Zealand."

This was a trip that had been on the back burner for a long time. It was to be our kind-of honeymoon, but there was no point in even thinking about going until I was well enough to face such a long flight.

"Lovely!" my sister said. "How exciting. You should go in March. I'll be in Australia for a wedding. You can just hop over from New Zealand and we'll meet up."

My girlfriend and I looked at each other.

"I don't know," I said. "If we should make any firm plans."

"Yeah, probably not," my girlfriend said. "Maybe we won't end up going. Not this year, anyway."

"Wow," my sister said. "I don't think I've ever seen two people less enthusiastic about booking a trip to New

Zealand. What's up? Is it a thing where one of you wants to go and the other doesn't?"

"No, I want to go," I said. "But I'm afraid that I'd be sick while I was there."

My sister looked at my girlfriend.

"Yeah, I totally want to go too," she said. "But I'm also afraid that Áine'd get sick."

"Sick?" my sister said. "Look at you, you're fine. Running around after us all week like a lunatic. There's nothing wrong with you."

"You're seeing me here. At home," I said. "With all my little gluten free foods, and all my little supplements and pills. Remember London? When I didn't have my DMSA? That's the kind of thing I'm talking about. What's the point of traveling half way across the world, and then lying around like a lump not being able to enjoy it?"

My sister looked at me like I was crazy.

"Then just bring along all your pills!" she said. "People get sick when they travel, they take a day in bed, and they get better. It's not a reason to stay home."

"I dunno," I said. "There's jet lag and everything..."

"Oh please," she said. "What's the time difference to New Zealand? Five or six hours? Going west, that's easy. I'm facing twelve hours between London and Australia, no matter which way I go. Don't sit there complaining to me about jet lag!"

"It's a long flight..." I said.

My sister rolled her eyes.

"But I was thinking," I continued. "That we could take the trip in stages. Stop in Hawaii for a few days so I could adjust."

"Hawaii!" my sister crowed. "Give me that laptop! Here, book it now! You're going to have the time of your life!"

We didn't book the trip right away, but my sister's enthusiasm was contagious. So what if 24 hours on a plane made my health crash? I could take a few days to lie in bed and recuperate, and when I was all together again, I'd be in New Zealand. In the summertime. It was the idea of skipping a month of winter that sold it to us in the end. Not having to live through January in New York State sounded like a miracle. We decided that we wouldn't attempt any side trips to Australia. We'd just fly in to Auckland at the end of December, fly out of Auckland three weeks later, and in between, take things easy and see as much of New Zealand as my health would permit. And on the way, we'd spend Christmas Day in Hawaii to break up the flight.

This plan sounded very realistic and do-able. I liked that it wasn't a high-pressure situation, where I had to perform, or I was destroying everything. My girlfriend had been to New Zealand before, so she didn't have her heart set on seeing every inch of the place. It was all right if we took things slowly.

Before we did the final booking of the flights, I found us a place to stay in Auckland that was very reasonably

189

priced. It was a little apartment that had a kitchenette, living room and even a laundry machine right there in the apartment. It sounded like an ideal place to spend four or five days holing up and getting myself together after the long flight. Then I sat my girlfriend down to ask her the most important question of all.

"What's the food like in New Zealand?"

"Just regular food," she said. "Like here."

I was worried about the gluten free angle. Traveling meant eating out every day. Would I be able to find cuisines that I knew were safe?

"Did you notice a lot of Indian restaurants when you were there?"

Most of the menu in every Indian restaurant was naturally gluten free.

"Well, I guess," she said. "In the cities. But a lot of towns were really small. One day I got stuck in this tiny place on Easter Sunday and literally nothing was open. I was starving. And then I found this gas station. Oh wow, it was great. They have surprisingly good food in gas stations in New Zealand, great little pies."

Pies were not going to help my situation.

"Okay," I said. "Then maybe we could stick to the big cities."

My girlfriend shook her head.

"That's not really how it works," she said. "I mean, all the cool stuff is kind of remote. The glacier, the fjords, the volcanic springs, they're not exactly in the middle of

Auckland, you know?"

"I know," I frowned.

"But really, don't worry," she said. "It's very easy to get around. The whole country is set up for tourists. It'll be no problem to figure this stuff out once we get there."

I went back to my computer and brought up Auckland on Google maps. I zoomed in and looked up and down the street that our hotel was on. I spotted a restaurant called Satya Indian Cuisine, clicked on their website, and sent them an email, asking if there were going to be open over the Christmas break. They replied, saying that they were, so I relaxed a little. I knew where I was going to be sleeping and what I was going to be eating for the first few days. It calmed me down enough to be able to go ahead and book the flights. I had six weeks to figure the rest of it out.

As soon as the flights were booked, something went wrong with my heart. Whenever I sat down, I could feel the thick, heavy sensation of blood pooling in my legs. It was as if the battery on my heart muscle was running low, and it couldn't pump the blood around my body at the normal speed. My hands were ghostly white and freezing and I began to have episodes where my teeth chattered and my body was wracked with shivers even if the room was toasty warm.

One of these episodes hit me right before our guests began to arrive for a party. A couple of weeks back, I had put out word that we were hosting a board game night for all the local lesbians. It had seemed like a great idea at the time. Kind of like the great idea of booking a month-long trip to the other side of the world with a dodgy heart. Some of the people who were coming were women I'd never met before. I'd hoped that our friendly invitation and warm welcome would impress them, but here I was, sitting forlornly on the couch, my teeth chattering and my arms jumping with shivers.

"Give me your feet," my girlfriend instructed.

She placed big red fluffy slippers on them.

"Now lie down," she said.

I lay on the couch, and she proceeded to roll me up in a comforter, and then top me off with three more blankets.

"Better?" she asked.

I nodded, and just then the doorbell rang.

"But I don't think I can get the door," I laughed.

"Stay right there," she said.

Two couples came in who I'd never met before. They introduced themselves to my girlfriend at the door, and then came into the living room and I extracted an arm from under all the blankets so that I could shake their hands.

"Are you all wrapped up because you're cold?" one of them asked.

The long answer to that question flashed through my head.

I've been chelating for a year and a half with Alpha Lipoic Acid, which you probably know as a heart antioxidant. I stopped taking it three weeks ago, and now my heart seems to have lost its ability to pump the blood around my body at the normal speed. The slow-moving blood isn't keeping me warm. I sincerely hope that this effect will pass before I have to take a flight to the other side of the world.

But I kept it brief. I said, "Yup, I'm freezing."

The evening went on, and I even shed the blankets during a lively game of Pictionary. But the whole episode made me doubt everything. Was it time to go back on ALA? Much to my relief, over the next few days, my heart slowly returned to normal and I decided I was okay.

And then it was my liver's turn. December seemed to be all about packages arriving in the mail. I had to make sure that I brought along a month's supply of each of my supplements on my trip. I also had to find a bottle of the only kind of sunblock I wasn't allergic to, which was devilishly hard to do in the middle of December. Then I'd ordered a clever product I'd found online, a little baggie made of silicone that was exactly the size of a slice of toast. When I went to New Zealand, I could bring along a loaf of gluten free bread, pop a slice in this baggie, and pop it in any toaster without fearing it would get contaminated with lingering gluten crumbs.

On top of all that, there were eight Hanukkah presents to buy, one for each night. The one I was most excited about was a pair of electronic dance mats for our exercise Playstation game Dance Dance Revolution. We had played it all the time before I got sick, and now that I was able to exercise a little again, I'd ordered the deluxe, padded version of the dance mats to optimize our game playing experience.

The dance mats arrived ready to assemble the same day that a surprise package arrived from my sister. It was a shiny new toaster. It made me laugh because she had teased us so much about our beat-up old toaster when she visited in the fall.

I called her up to thank her.

"We're not throwing the old one away," I laughed. "We're going to keep it for gluten toast. Gluten won't be banished to the oven anymore. And the new one will be all mine, gluten free!"

Since my girlfriend wasn't home, I went down to the basement to assemble the dance mats. There were pieces of stiff foam that needed to be fit together like puzzle pieces and then zipped up inside the dance mats. The foam had a strong chemical smell, and I washed my hands thoroughly when I was done, but the damage was already done.

"Hey, a new toaster!" my girlfriend exclaimed when she got home.

"Stupid toaster," I said. "We don't need a new one."

I felt nauseous, headachy, and very cranky. I'd felt like this back during the dump phase, whenever I'd gone into stores that had a lot of products that smelled like chemicals. The dollar store where we'd lived before had been particularly bad. Our home was usually free of chemical crap, but now that it had invaded my space, I'd been instantly wiped out.

A wave of despair washed over me and tears began to leak out of my eyes. If I couldn't deal with opening a couple of simple holiday gifts, how was I supposed to travel? I'd set up my life in a gluten-free chemical-free bubble. How was I supposed to function in the real world? I was kidding myself if I thought that I was well. I was still sick as dog.

The despair died down over the next day or so, and was followed by a vicious bout of constipation, which was a sure sign that my liver was struggling. It made sense. ALA was as much an antioxidant for the liver as it was for the heart.

Trying out the new toaster brought on another liver episode, and that was followed by another when I presented the dance mats to my girlfriend on the first night of Hanukkah and we tried them out.

The next morning, my girlfriend found me dragging the mats out to the garage.

"What are you doing?" she asked.

"I'm not going to have them in this house!" I said in an angry fit of tears.

"But you just gave them to me," my girlfriend said. "When can I have them back?"

"Never!" I said. "I'm going to go online and sell them!"

❧❦

My hip went out the next day when I bent down to tie my shoe. This hadn't happened to me in more than six months, not since we'd moved to Beacon. I'd been sure that chelation had cleared this up permanently. I sat down and rested for a few minutes, still feeling the pain even as I sat. The pain went on and on, and I was afraid to stand in case I made things much worse. I was stranded in a chair that was far away from the TV or a bookshelf. I had nothing to do except think.

What was I going to do now? We were due to leave on our trip in a week. I hadn't needed the services of a chiropractor since we'd moved to our new home. Did it make more sense to drive for an hour to the guy by our old home, or try to find a new one here? The old guy had been good, but when my right hip was out, driving was very hard, lifting my foot from the gas to the brake hurt like hell. Maybe my girlfriend would drive me there.

While I thought, I idly examined my nails, and was surprised to find them all dotted with white horizontal lines. The Mee's Lines were back, the classic badge of heavy metal toxicity that I'd unknowingly worn throughout childhood.

196

The words of my old chiropractor suddenly echoed through my head.

Pour enough antioxidants down someone's throat, and they're sure to feel fine for a while. But what happens when you stop?

Well here I was, going cold turkey on the antioxidants, and it looked like every one of my mercury symptoms was popping up to make a reappearance. What did it mean? Had ALA just been a trick, a coat of paint thrown onto a moldy wall? Now that it was wearing away, was the nastiness that had been there all along beginning to show through?

My hip pain faded without the help of a chiropractor, and I vacillated back and forth, thinking one day that the smartest thing to do would be to take some stupid ALA, deciding the next that I didn't need to, that all of the symptoms I was experiencing were passing temporary blips.

And then it was two days before my trip, and I was sitting in a coffee shop, having a last cup of peppermint tea with my friend Kelly.

I was complaining bitterly about the exhaustive preparations I'd had to make for a trip I'd lost all enthusiasm for.

"And I bought a little baggie for my gluten free bread that can go in toasters. But after the first week when I eat up the loaf of bread I bring, I don't know what I'm going to eat. I haven't been feeling great, so I didn't have enough time to do all the research I wanted to. I didn't even get to look up if they have gluten free bread in New Zealand. Or if they even let you bring bread through customs."

Kelly's brow was creased.

"Let's back up," she said. "To the plastic bag you're going to put in a toaster?"

"It's not plastic," I said. "It's silicone, and the heat goes through it, but it protects the bread from contamination by gluten crumbs left in the toaster."

"I see what you mean," she said. "You bought a toast condom."

"Well, yes," I said. "I guess I did."

"And you're dreading spending a month in Hawaii and New Zealand because there's a possibility you might get sick."

"I know I sound like a real whiner," I said. "But you didn't know me when I was really sick. The six months I've been living here, it's the first time I've ever felt properly healthy. I'm afraid I'll lose that if I leave. What if it only works here?"

"Health isn't something that exists in a place," Kelly said. "It goes wherever you go. It's in your body."

"I guess," I said. "But I feel like I'm standing in line for one of those crazy big rollercoasters at Six Flags. Everyone around me is saying how much fun it's going to be, but I'm afraid it's just going to make me throw up."

"Well, I'd be happy to help," Kelly said. "I can go ahead and take your place on the trip, and you can stay here and shovel the snow and feed my cats."

I began to smile, and then to laugh.

"I'm going to have a good time?" I said.

"That's why you're going," Kelly said. "Right?"

My final day of packing and preparation was marred by pretty dramatic PMS. Folding my shorts and t-shirts and packing them in my bag, tears kept leaking from my eyes. But when it got to the point when we finally left the house, it was as if a great weight was taken from my shoulders. I didn't have to prepare anymore. I didn't have to keep guessing what was going to happen, preparing for every possible outcome. I just had to do it, live through it, and enjoy it if I could.

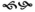

Five days later, I was putting my laundry in the washing machine in the little apartment I'd found online in Auckland. The night before, we'd eaten our dinner at the Indian restaurant I'd found on Google maps, and just a few hours ago, we'd eaten our lunch at a nearby burger joint that had a full gluten free menu. Then we'd stopped in the bookstore to buy the *Rough Guide to New Zealand*.

I picked it up now, and studied the maps and lists of attractions. This was something I hadn't had a single spare moment to do during all of my extensive preparations. Turning to the section on the north island, I learned that just a couple hours away, there was a place where you could take a boat trip through a cave filled with glowworms. Not far from there in Rotorua, there were baths build around volcanic hot springs, and state parks that were filled with bubbling mud pools and alien yellow and green sulfuric formations.

We were slated to spend another three days in Auckland so that I could recover, but I was beginning to wonder what exactly I needed to recover from. The flight to Hawaii had been uneventful. The hotel there, the 80 degree heat, and Christmas Day on the beach had been glorious. Then the dreaded overnight flight to Auckland had been fine. I'd even slept for a few hours by taking a sleeping pill, one that I'd practiced taking at home to make sure I wouldn't have a bad reaction to it. Our first day in Auckland, I'd been out of sorts and cranky, but now I was raring to go.

"Let's check out early," I said to my girlfriend. "And go see the glowworms tomorrow. Then head to Rotorua."

"Are you sure?" she asked. "You're okay?"

"Perfect," I said.

I found an internet café and looked up gluten free dining options in Rotorua. There were much better than your average American town of that size. Besides an Indian restaurant, there was a branch of the burger joint with the gluten free menu, and also a branch of a pizza place with a full gluten free menu. It looked like this was going to be pretty easy.

We went to the tourist office to book our travel and

accommodation. We booked three nights in Rotorua.

"What happens after that?" I asked my girlfriend.

"We'll just move on to the next place the looks good," my girlfriend said. "We don't have to plan it all right now."

And so we played it by ear, booking buses, flights, tours, ferries as we went. We stayed in accommodations that had kitchenettes when we could, and I had plenty of opportunities to use the toast condom. When the loaf of bread I brought along ran out, I bought more gluten free bread in the supermarket across the road from our B&B. Their gluten free selection was far better than that of most American supermarkets.

We saw the glowworms in their cave, a luminous green constellation hanging eerily from above. We saw the steam rise off the pools of water heated by the lava just under the surface of the earth. We took nature tours, saw kiwi fruit growing on the vine, and kiwi birds in the darkened houses where they were raised before being released into the wild. We took a boat out into a craggy fjord, so tall that waterfalls that began at the top disappeared into mist before they reached the bottom.

And I walked. I hiked. I dragged my luggage around with me for three weeks. I got up every day and went out and saw everything and did everything. And then I got up and did it all again the next day. I even climbed a mountain. It wasn't much of a mountain by Kiwi standards, but sitting at the top of it, eating an apple while my girlfriend took pictures of me and the incredible scenery, I felt like I'd climbed to the top of the world.

I wasn't the same person that I'd been six months or a year before. A profound change had taken place inside me. I felt clarity, peace, resilience, strength. And under it all, there was a bedrock of knowing, a sureness that I could rely on this. My body was no longer struggling, crushed under an unbearable burden. The mercury was gone, I had finally entered a space of true healing.

❧

Epilogue

It's hard not to brag. It's been over a year since I came home from New Zealand, and it's been a year of astonishing good health. While I chelated, all my hope was pinned on one goal: getting myself back to the state of health I'd enjoyed right before I got my amalgams removed.

What I never expected, what I never dreamed possible, was that I would surpass that goal.

When I came home from that trip, I knew that I'd moved to a whole other level. Chelation, and my alarming cold-turkey reaction to quitting antioxidants, were behind me. I'd achieved a far more stable state of being. But what was this state like? What were the boundaries of my abilities now?

I knew I could hike and climb a mountain, but what else could I do? Could I run? I went to the gym and got on a treadmill and jogged for 20 minutes without a problem. Could I eat sugar? Was the candida gone? I experimented by eating a little maple syrup, and then trying out some chocolate. The candida rash I got was minimal, but it was still there. I was happy to see that my negative reaction to the caffeine had disappeared, it no longer kept me up at night to eat a little chocolate. But I decided to play it safe and still avoid sugar.

And the big question—could I eat gluten? I tried a handful of goldfish crackers, and found that I had the very mild neuropathy in my scalp and fingers just like last time. Even after a course of NAET, a kind of acupuncture specially designed to curb allergies, I still reacted to gluten in a very mild way. I decided to stay gluten free until my reaction disappeared completely.

My disappointment about my limitations was very short-lived because I had gained the most important thing of all. My brain was now permanently functional and fog-free, my emotions were balanced. My habitual, unconscious approach to life shifted to a place of contentment and optimism. I didn't struggle with my emotions anymore. I felt calm most of the time, and when thorny emotional issues came up, I navigated them with aplomb.

This didn't mean that I felt completely happy every moment. It was more that my emotional reactions to things stopped being weighted down by a load of mercury gloom. My negative feelings were now in proportion to the events that caused them, making them so much easier to manage.

And because my inner emotional landscape changed, my words and actions changed too. It wasn't very dramatic, it wasn't like I became a whole other person. But the way that I was responding to life now was something that I'd often seen in others, and had been frankly envious of. I found myself automatically acting like an emotionally resilient person, something I'd always tried to emulate, but had never experienced from the inside. I cried a lot less. I was harder to offend. I didn't spend a lot of time fretting about what people 'really meant' if they made an odd comment about me. Everything was just easier, on a day by day, and on a minute by minute basis.

And most importantly of all, harmony reigned in my relationship. It wasn't like my girlfriend and I never fought. We disagreed vehemently over issues like everyone else. But now our lines of communication were clear. They weren't burdened with the anxiety and misunderstandings caused by mercury. When she and I disagreed, we went ahead and argued, we resolved it, we got over it and got on with our lives.

Healing is of course, an ongoing process. It took me 32 years to get as sick as I did, and though I'm healthier now than I've ever been in my life, I'm not resting on my laurels. The heavy metal mess isn't quite cleaned up yet.

Though I've finished my mercury chelation, I still do ongoing rounds of DMSA to reduce my burden of lead. Most of the lead in my body is stored in my bones, and will only come out slowly over a period of years as I chelate it. Thankfully, DMSA is presenting none of the hardships it did the first time around. I'm prepared this time, keeping firm control over my yeast issues.

Nowadays, besides avoiding sugar and gluten, I can eat

whatever I want. I also take a lot fewer supplements than I did when I was on ALA. In the past year, I dropped the ones I no longer need: B12, inositol, digestive enzymes, progesterone cream, kelp, Adrenal Cortex, chromium, glutamine. But because I'm chelating, and still technically heavy metal toxic, I still take the basics: Vitamin C, vitamin E, flax oil, magnesium, milk thistle and ginkgo biloba. I also take probiotics, to help keep me free of yeast symptoms.

Yeast and gluten intolerance are my only two symptoms that still linger. I do hope that they will fade away as my body burden of lead decreases. I would like to make it all the way to 100% perfect health some day. But if this never happens, I won't complain. I've been given more than I could ever have dreamed. My life is full of love, friendship, work, cats, creativity, and the thing that makes it all possible: stable, beautiful health.

Acknowledgements

꿍

The author would like to thank Sunshine for his feedback on portions of this manuscript, and also the Beacon Women's Writing Group for their feedback and support.

Special thanks to Kelly Kingman and Susan Walsh for their design and publishing advice.

And super-extra-special thanks to Nora for letting me write about such a difficult time in our relationship, and for being the best partner a mercury toxic girl could ever wish for.

꿍

To read more mercury stories, and to find out more about the resources mentioned in this book, go to: www.mercurystories.com.

Lightning Source UK Ltd.
Milton Keynes UK
UKOW02f2330150816

280781UK00001B/20/P